Pregnancy & birth
The essential checklists

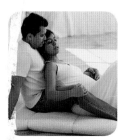
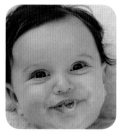
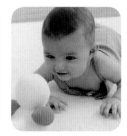

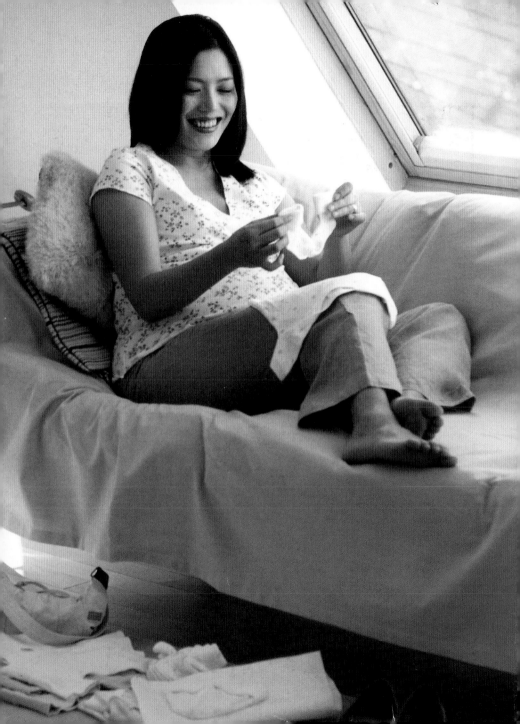

Pregnancy
& birth
The essential checklists

Karen Sullivan

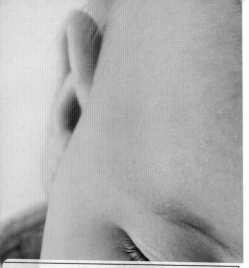

London, New York, Munich, Melbourne, Delhi

Project Editor Angela Baynham
Designer Hannah Moore
Senior Editor Helen Murray
Senior Art Editor Liz Sephton
Picture Librarian Romaine Werblow
Production Editor Kelly Salih
Senior Production Editor Jenny Woodcock
Production Controller Mandy Inness
Creative Technical Support Sonia Charbonnier
Managing Editor Penny Warren
Managing Art Editor Glenda Fisher
Category Publisher Peggy Vance

First published in Great Britain in 2009 by
Dorling Kindersley Limited
80 Strand, London WC2R ORL

Penguin Group (UK)

A CIP catalogue record for this book is available from the British Library.

ISBN: 978-1-4053-4670-2

Printed and bound in China by
Hung Hing Printing Group Ltd

Discover more at
www.dk.com

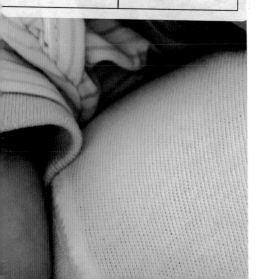

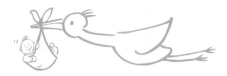

Contents

Introduction

Whether having a baby is part of your long-term plans, or an unexpected surprise, becoming pregnant is an emotionally charged, life-changing event. And as the hormones begin to surge through your body, you find yourself faced with the daunting task of juggling pregnancy and work, planning the birth, and preparing for your new life with a baby. There is a bewildering array of choices to think about and arrangements to be made, not to mention getting to grips with the concept of becoming a mum.

But help is to hand. This indispensable little book will ease you through the process of organizing your life, helping you to sail through pregnancy, plan the birth you want, and deal with day-to-day life with your newborn. You'll find tips for everything from common health issues, arranging and decorating your baby's nursery, and purchasing essential equipment, to planning your birth and choosing the best birth options and pain relief, selecting the right childbirth classes, planning for childcare, coping with pregnancy and new motherhood while at work, and bathing your new baby and encouraging her to sleep.

We'll look at how to stretch your budget to accommodate your new arrival, your rights and benefits during pregnancy, and what to expect from the healthcare system at every stage. You'll find logs for charting your baby's sleep and feeding patterns and her growth and development, and vital information to ensure that your baby is happy, healthy, and stimulated. We'll look at travelling and transportation, packing the perfect hospital bag, keeping your handbag topped up with pregnancy essentials, and what your baby needs in her changing bag. I'll also provide you with an at-a-glance list of symptoms that confirm you are in labour, and a handy checklist for your birth partner, too.

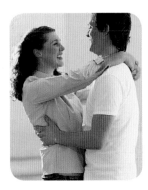
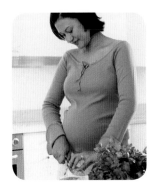
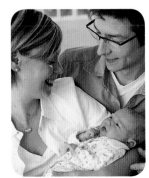

Once your baby is here, I'll talk you through the early days of feeding, dealing with everything from breastfeeding problems and support to preparing those first bottles, and even weaning. I'll lead you through the immunization schedule, common health issues and teething, and the processes of registering your baby's birth and arranging for her first passport. I'll also help you to choose the perfect toys and games to keep your baby contented and entertained at each stage during her first year.

Whether you are a first-time mum-to-be, or a seasoned expert, this book will be very useful. Its handy checklist format allows you to see at a glance what exactly is needed in any circumstance or situation, which allows you to use your precious time wisely, ticking off the essentials as you move through the months and keep on top of what needs to be plotted, planned, and purchased. What's more, there is space allowed at the end of every checklist for you to add your own ideas and details, making each list even more relevant and personal to you and your baby.

Pregnancy & Birth: The Essential Checklists will not only help you to stay on top of things, but it will keep you one step ahead, leaving you with all the time you need for the things that really matter.

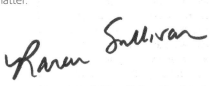

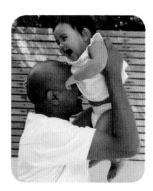 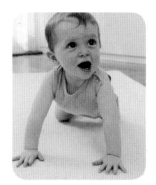 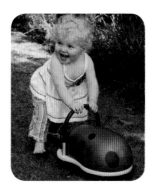

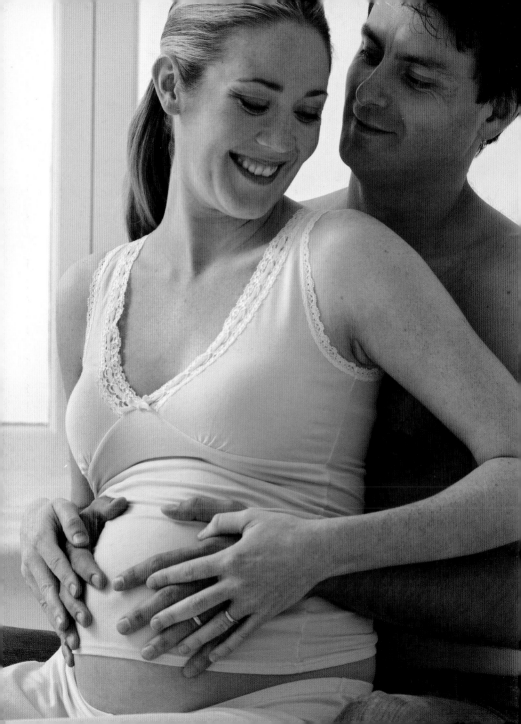

Pregnancy

What to do if the test is positive

The confirmation that you are about to become a mother heralds a new stage in your life, and now is the perfect time to start planning and preparing for the changes ahead. You may be experiencing mixed feelings about the news, and that's entirely normal. Beginning the preparations can help you to come to terms with your new status.

○ **Take a second test**: although modern pregnancy tests are very accurate, they sometimes get it wrong

○ **Make an appointment to see your GP** – he or she will need to begin the booking-in procedure

○ **Let your doctor know if your immunizations are not up to date**

○ **Avoid taking new medication**, and consult your doctor if you need to take any regular medication

○ **Calculate your estimated delivery date** (see box, opposite)

○ **If you aren't already taking folic acid, start now**, as this is essential for your new baby's development

○ **Cut out alcohol and cigarettes**, which have been linked to health problems in babies

○ **Develop a healthy eating plan** (see pages 18–19), with plenty of fresh fruits and vegetables, lean proteins, good-quality carbs, and foods rich in iron and folic acid

○ **Exercise moderately** – keeping fit helps to ensure an easier pregnancy and birth (see pages 28–29)

○ **If you usually drink coffee, cut back** or try decaffeinated coffee or herbal tea instead; a little caffeine won't hurt your baby, but caffeine has been linked to miscarriage in some women

○ **Listen to your body**: if you are tired, take a nap; if you are hungry, have a snack – the very best way to overcome and cope with the symptoms of pregnancy is to listen and respond to your body's signals

○ **Share the news** – some women like to wait until they've seen a scan, or passed the 12-week mark, but there's no reason why you can't tell a few people your good news now

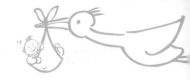

- **Make sure you have a good support network** of friends, family, and your partner, as well as your doctor and/or midwife, who can answer the multitude of questions that are likely to crop up during the coming months

- **Join an online community of pregnant women** and new mums who can share advice and stories

- **Start a pregnancy diary**, noting down how you are feeling, what symptoms you are experiencing, and any hopes or plans you have for the months to come; ask your partner or a friend to take a photo of you every month to keep track of your changing body

- **Invest in a few pregnancy books** to keep tabs on what's happening to your baby – and you!

- **Look around for good antenatal classes** – although you are unlikely to begin these for several months, they often get booked up well in advance

- **Sign up for daily pregnancy updates via email** – these are based on your estimated due date; good ones to try include www.pregnancy.about.com and www.babycentre.co.uk

- **Enjoy your pregnancy**

- ....

- ....

- ....

Your estimated due date

This date is calculated by adding seven days to the first day of your last menstrual period, and then subtracting three months. So, if your last period was on 1 February, your baby will arrive somewhere around 8 November. Some experts believe that caucasian first-time mums should add an extra 15 days to this date; however, your first scan will pinpoint an accurate date.

Appointments, tests, and scans

Once your pregnancy is confirmed, you will be regularly monitored to ensure that both you and your baby are healthy. These are exciting times, full of anticipation, concerns, and huge changes to your body. Your antenatal appointments, tests, and scans will provide you with an opportunity to ask questions and get the reassurance you need.

Routine antenatal appointments

For a first baby, you will have an appointment with your doctor or midwife at:

- ○ **8–10 weeks** – booking-in appointment
- ○ **16 weeks**
- ○ **25 weeks**
- ○ **28 weeks**
- ○ **31 weeks**
- ○ **36 weeks**
- ○ **38 weeks**
- ○ **40 weeks**
- ○ **41 weeks** – assuming you haven't had your baby by then

If you have already had a baby, and have an uncomplicated pregnancy, you should have seven antenatal appointments: the booking-in visit, and then checks at about 16, 28, 34, 36, 38, and 41 weeks.

Blood tests

At the booking-in appointment, a small sample of your blood will be tested for:

- ○ **Your blood group**
- ○ **Your rhesus status** – whether you have a positive or negative blood group
- ○ **HIV**
- ○ **Hepatitis B**
- ○ **Rubella immunity**
- ○ **Red blood cell abnormalities**, such as sickle cell disease

Scans

Most women have two scans, although you may be offered more if you have a high-risk pregnancy; you may also be scanned later in your pregnancy to check the size and   of your baby or placenta. Otherwise, expect scans at:

○ **10–14 weeks** – to confirm your due date and detect twins; to check nuchal translucency (NT) to assess the risk of Down's syndrome

○ **18–20 weeks** – to check your baby is developing properly, and that the placenta is in a safe position

Screening tests

○ **11–14 weeks** – the combined test, which involves an NT scan (see above) and blood tests to check for chemicals that could indicate conditions such as spina bifida or Down's syndrome, among others

Diagnostic tests

○ **Urine tests** will be done at every appointment to check for the presence of protein (which could indicate pre-eclampsia), urinary tract infections, and sugar (which could indicate gestational diabetes)

○ **Blood pressure** is checked at every appointment to ensure that it doesn't rise significantly, as this could be a sign of pre-eclampsia

If screening tests suggest that your baby has a high risk of Down's syndrome or other chromosomal abnormalities, you may be offered:

○ **Chorionic villus sampling (CVS)**, in which tiny samples of the chorionic villi (finger-like projections on the placenta) are taken to check the genetic information they carry:

  ○ Transvaginal CVS is done at 11–13 weeks, when a small tube or a pair of forceps is inserted through your cervix

  ○ Transabdominal CVS is usually done after 13 weeks, when a needle is inserted through your abdomen into your placenta

○ **Amniocentesis**, in which a needle is inserted into your womb and amniotic fluid is removed for testing); this is done after 14 weeks

○ _____

○ _____

Budgeting for baby

Early pregnancy is a great time to look closely at your financial situation and plan ahead. There's no doubt that having a baby can be expensive, but with a little tweaking of the budget, and some prudent cuts, you can help to make sure that you are in a suitably stable financial position to enjoy life as a parent.

- ○ **Work out how much you spend each month** (include all regular outgoings)
- ○ **Consider swapping service providers for better deals**
- ○ **Consider paying utility bills by direct debit**, or make a note on the calendar for "early payment discount" dates; both can save you a lot of money
- ○ **Check your bank statements** to be sure that your standing orders and direct debits are correct, up to date, and necessary
- ○ **Take a look at your credit card spending**; if you've maxed out your cards, it might be a good idea to get a single loan to repay them, which will have a better rate of interest with more manageable monthly payments
- ○ **Work out income and expenditure** based on income you will be receiving while you are on maternity leave – check out websites that help you do this and work out what disposable income you'll have left over
- ○ **Plan as though you have less income than you expect**, which will give you some flexibility if you decide to go back to work a little later than planned, or if you decide to work fewer hours on your return
- ○ **Check that you are getting all the benefits** to which you are entitled
- ○ **Childcare may be your single greatest cost** when raising your baby; investigate tax credits, help for working mums, and childcare vouchers that might be available from the government
- ○ **Consider your car**: you are going to need something practical and reliable – if you have a two-seater, for example, you'll need a larger car – look around for a good secondhand car as new cars lose their value quickly
- ○ **Start putting a little money aside each month** to use after your baby is born; even a few pounds a month will quickly accumulate and make a difference

- **Add up the estimated costs of "running" your baby** – include childcare, babysitting, nappies, formula (if you don't intend to breastfeed), baby equipment and clothes, baby toiletries, and toys and books
- **Buy one key item for your baby each month**, to spread the cost
- **Register big items**, such as your baby's cot, pushchair, and car seat, on a "wish list" at a good department store, so that friends and family can club together and get you what you need (see page 78)
- **Remember that the most expensive** items are not necessarily the best
- **Don't be proud**! Ask family and friends with older children to lend you secondhand equipment or clothes, and visit nearly new sales or eBay
- ....
- ....
- ....

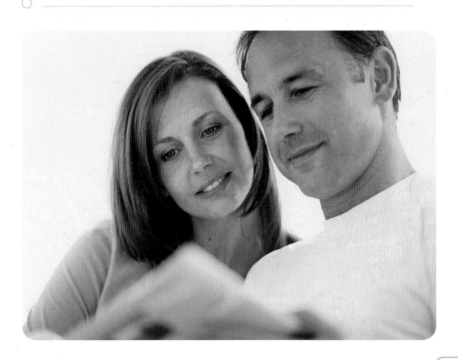

Your basic maternity wardrobe

While pregnancy is a great opportunity to purchase a new wardrobe, it's worth cutting corners wherever you can. For one thing, you'll be so sick of your maternity clothes by the end of your pregnancy, they may never be worn again. Here are some great ideas for dressing well – and on a budget.

○ **Think about the seasons when you are shopping**, so you don't end up with a collection of long-sleeved maternity tops if you'll be heavily pregnant in summer

○ **Start with a few items and add pieces as you need them** – aim to buy one or two new items every month throughout pregnancy to keep reviving your maternity wardrobe

○ **For the office, purchase a few pieces** of neutral, simply shaped basic garments, and accessorize them with scarves and jewellery

○ **Don't hesitate to accept offers of maternity clothes** from friends and relatives; wearing these clothes at home will leave you with a little more money to spend on clothes for work

○ **Keep your own style and comfort level in mind** – if you weren't comfortable wearing dresses or smart jackets before your pregnancy, you are unlikely to be so now

○ **Buy quality, feel-good clothes** – you are going to be wearing these a lot

○ **Invest in two good-quality maternity bras**, and don't be surprised if they need to be replaced in a few months' time

○ **Maternity underwear is an unnecessary expense** – just buy a larger size; however, this doesn't apply to other maternity clothing, which is specially designed to accommodate your growing bump

○ **It's worth investing in a good pair of maternity trousers** – something stretchy, with an adjustable waist; or choose low-slung trousers that can sit neatly under your growing bump

○ **If you've got an old pair of jeans** that are ready for recycling, cut out the front, and sew in an elasticated panel

○ **Raid your partner's cupboard** – large T-shirts or dress shirts and cardies can be ruched in with a low-slung belt to create comfortable maternity wear that doesn't impact on your budget

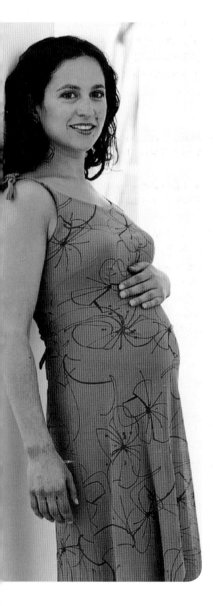

○ **Empire-cut dresses** will see you through most of your pregnancy

○ **You can purchase a "belly band"**, which is designed to fill the gap between shirts or tops and trousers, as your waist expands

○ **Don't forget your shoes** – your centre of gravity changes when you are pregnant as your weight shifts forward, and high heels can be dangerous (not to mention uncomfortable); look for elegant flats or shoes with a low heel

○ **In the summer**, go for clothing made of natural fabrics, such as linen and cotton; loose-cut dresses and trousers, and flowing skirts and tops will help you to stay cool

○ **Think twice before investing in a winter coat** – you are likely to feel very warm towards the end of your pregnancy, and may find it more comfortable to wear plenty of layered knits rather than one coat or jacket

○ ....

○ ....

○ ....

○ ....

Nutrition during pregnancy

By now you'll be aware that what you eat is very important during pregnancy. A healthy diet not only helps to ensure that your baby gets all the nutrients he needs for optimum growth and development, but it will also minimize the risk of pregnancy complications, and provide you with plenty of energy. Your healthy pregnancy diet should include:

○ **Wholegrains**, such as wholemeal bread and pasta, brown rice, pulses, and grains (such as barley, oats, and quinoa), to provide a sustained source of energy, plenty of fibre (see opposite), and essential B vitamins

○ **Good sources of calcium**, to ensure the healthy development of your baby's bones and teeth – you'll find calcium in dairy products, soya products, leafy green vegetables, and some fish

○ **Folic acid**, for your baby's nervous system; look for it in dark green vegetables, nuts, and wholegrains

○ **Protein**, which is necessary for the development of every new cell in your baby's body – good-quality protein is found in pulses, wholegrains, nuts, soya, dairy produce, eggs, lean meats, poultry, and fish

○ **Vitamin C**, which not only helps your body to fight infection, and maximizes the absorption of iron, but is also essential for the growth of a strong placenta – fresh fruit and vegetables provide plenty of iron

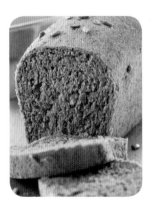
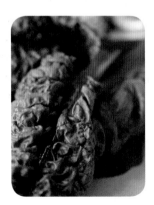
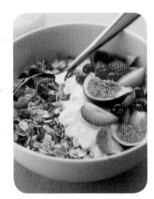

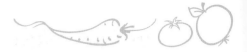

- **Iron-rich foods**, which help to prevent anaemia, and ensure that your baby builds up adequate iron stores; try lean red meats, leafy green vegetables, fish, dried fruits, beetroot, wholegrain bread, and iron-fortified cereals
- **Fibre**, to ensure that nutrients are efficiently absorbed, and your bowel movements are regular – wholegrains should give you plenty
- **Essential fatty acids**, which are necessary for your baby's development, particularly his nervous system, brain, and vision – good sources include eggs, nuts, seeds, and cold-water oily fish (such as salmon and mackerel)
- **Fresh water**, to keep you and your baby well hydrated

- _____
- _____
- _____

Foods to avoid during pregnancy

- **Liver and cod liver oil** – these can provide too much of the animal form of vitamin A, which is linked to birth defects
- **Meat pâtés**, which can contain food-borne illnesses
- **Unpasteurized soft or blue cheese**, such as Camembert, goat's cheese, Brie, and Stilton – these can contain listeria
- **Raw or partially cooked eggs**, as these can contain salmonella
- **Raw or undercooked meat, fish, and poultry** – these can contain salmonella or *Toxoplasma gondii*, which can cause toxoplasmosis
- **Ready-to-eat salads in bags** because of the risk of listeria
- **Too much oily fish**, which can contain pollutants such as dioxins, mercury, and PCBs; stick to two servings per week

- _____
- _____
- _____

Perfect pregnancy snacks

Not only does your blood sugar have a tendency to dip and soar during pregnancy, leaving you feeling tired and lethargic, but your body needs regular refuelling to keep up with the demands placed upon it. Treat your snacks as "mini meals": they should be balanced and contain plenty of essential nutrients (see pages 18–19), with no empty calories.

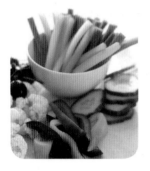

Great snack ideas include:

- ○ Nuts or seeds
- ○ Plain live yogurt with fresh fruit
- ○ Fresh fruit and vegetables with dips
- ○ Toast with nut butters or high-fruit spreads
- ○ Fruit smoothies
- ○ Vegetable soup
- ○ Dried fruit
- ○ Good-quality, low-sugar muesli bars
- ○ Cheese sticks
- ○ Small sandwiches with plenty of salad
- ○ Pasta or cous cous salads, with lots of veggies
- ○ Wholegrain, unsweetened breakfast cereal
- ○ Hardboiled eggs
- ○ ....
- ○ ....

Bedtime snacks

Have a snack before bed to help you sleep and to ensure you don't wake up with hunger pains. Go for turkey, eggs, dairy produce, and tuna, which are great sources of the amino acid tryptophan, which encourages restful sleep.

Your pregnancy handbag

Stocking up your handbag with everything you need to deal with pregnancy symptoms and the daily reality of being pregnant on the go will help to ensure that you are prepared for any eventuality. Useful items include:

- ○ **Sanitary towels**, for spotting or leaking
- ○ **A plastic or lined paper bag**, in the event that you are sick while out
- ○ **A travel toothbrush** (in the event that vomiting catches you unawares)
- ○ **A small spray bottle of water**, for when you experience flushes
- ○ **Bottled water** to keep you and your baby hydrated
- ○ **Cream or lotion** for dry skin or itching
- ○ **Wet wipes** for freshening up
- ○ **Your doctor's and midwife's phone numbers**
- ○ **Details of an emergency contact**, in the event that you become unwell and help is required
- ○ **Rescue Remedy or Emergency Essence** for sudden anxiety or stress
- ○ **Healthy snacks** to keep blood-sugar levels steady, and to ease nausea
- ○ **A suitable antacid**
- ○ ....
- ○ ....
- ○ ....

When to take extra care

If you carry an extra pair of shoes in your pregnancy handbag, make sure you wrap them in a plastic bag to prevent the spread of micro-organisms picked up from the ground. Always rinse out your water bottle before refilling it to prevent bacterial growth, and get rid of any used tissues, which can harbour germs.

Maternity rights and benefits

There are strict guidelines for employees to follow that support your rights as an employee during pregnancy and once your baby is born, and you will also be entitled to a variety of benefits. It's a good idea to investigate what's on offer, so that you know where you stand.

Maternity leave and pay

- **Women in the UK are entitled to 52 weeks' maternity leave** (statutory maternity leave or SML), plus any unused holiday leave; you will also accrue holiday leave over the 52-week period, which can be added on to the end

- **You must take a minimum of two weeks' leave** after the birth of your baby – or four weeks if you work in a factory

- **The SML period is made up of 26 weeks'** ordinary maternity leave (OML) followed immediately by 26 weeks' additional maternity leave (AML)

- **Statutory maternity pay (SMP)** is paid for the first 39 weeks of maternity leave; you will qualify if you:
  - Have been employed for at least 26 weeks, extending into the 15th week before the week your baby is due
  - Earn at least £95 a week
  - Have provided your employer with medical evidence of your pregnancy (a MATB1 form, issued in your 21st week of pregnancy) at least 15 weeks before your baby is due
  - Have given 28 days' notice of the date from which you want to start your SMP

- **SMP is payable at a rate of 90 per cent** of your average weekly earnings (there is no upper limit) for the first six weeks; the remaining 33 weeks are paid at either the standard weekly rate, or 90 per cent of your average weekly earnings, if this is lower

- **If you don't qualify for SMP**, you may qualify for Maternity Allowance (MA) – see your local benefits office for details

- **You must not work during your SML**, although you are allowed 10 "keeping in touch" days within that period

Benefits during leave

○ **It's important to check your contract** and the company maternity policy to understand which benefits continue throughout your maternity leave. However, you will continue to receive your statutory annual leave entitlement, which is currently 28 days (including bank holidays) for a full 52 weeks off

○ **While you are on maternity leave**, your company must continue to contribute to any occupational pension scheme you have in place

Enhanced maternity leave

○ **Your employer may offer a package** outside the statutory system, including:

   ○ A higher percentage of your income paid during leave

   ○ More than 52 weeks' leave

   ○ A guarantee of your old job back if you return within three years

Rights

○ **You are entitled to paid time off** for antenatal care

○ **Particular health and safety rules apply** (see page 25)

○ **You are protected against unfair treatment**

○ **Your employer can't change your terms and conditions of employment** while you're pregnant without your agreement

○ _____

○ _____

Antenatal time off

You are not only entitled to time off at full pay to attend antenatal appointments, but you may also take paid time off for antenatal classes and anything else your doctor or midwife suggest is required for a healthy pregnancy and delivery.

Your pregnancy at work toolkit

Being prepared to deal with any pregnancy symptoms during working hours can help you to feel on the ball, and to remain professional with the minimum amount of fuss. You may like to include:

- ○ **Bottles of fresh water** to stay hydrated and alert
- ○ **Decaf or herbal tea**
- ○ **Healthy snacks** to keep you going (see page 20)
- ○ **Natural remedies** for headaches, heartburn, and nausea (see pages 36–37)
- ○ **A cushion, heating pad, or hot water bottle** for backache
- ○ **A footstool to keep your feet up** (under your desk, of course)
- ○ **An alarm clock**, in case you manage to catch a few winks in your break
- ○ **A toothbrush and toothpaste**, to help recovery from vomiting episodes
- ○ **A notebook** listing ongoing projects and their status
- ○ **Your job description**, highlighting your regular routines and tasks
- ○ **A list of everyone you work with**, and their contact details
- ○ **A master list of file names and locations** on your computer, with a password set up to access all personal files
- ○ _____
- ○ _____
- ○ _____

Rest and recharge

Take extra breaks now and then to recharge your batteries if you need to, but make sure you keep up with your work and maintain a professional manner to set the standard for how people treat you and your pregnancy.

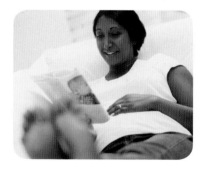

Hazards at work

It is completely safe to continue working in most jobs and companies while pregnant. However, it is important to be aware of any potential risks to you and/or your baby. If your job involves any of the situations listed below, you are within your legal rights to ask for changes to be made to your job description and working practice.

○ **Working with animals**, which may carry *E. coli* or organisms that cause tularaemia, toxoplasmosis, or histoplasmosis

○ **Working with chemicals**, such as those used in medical, dental, or pharmaceutical occupations, as well as in painting, cleaning, farming, dry-cleaning, gardening, pest-control, and carpet-cleaning

○ **Exposure to food hazards**, such as listeria, *E. coli*, and salmonella, which can be encountered by handling raw foods

○ **Exposure to secondhand smoke**, which crosses the placental barrier and increases the level of carbon monoxide in your baby's developing brain

○ **Exposure to radiation**, from x-rays

○ **Exposure to viral hazards**, in medical settings or even childcare facilities, where you may be in contact with viruses that may harm your baby

○ **Requirement to do heavy lifting**

○ **Working long hours spent standing or sitting**

○ **Working excessive hours**

○ **Working in awkward spaces and work stations**

○ **Working under stress**, an excess of which has now been linked to low birth weight, high blood pressure, and developmental and behaviour problems in your baby

○ **Exposure to violence**

○ **Wearing a tight-fitting uniform**, which can make you uncomfortable and exacerbate pregnancy symptoms

○ ....

○ ....

○ ....

Travelling during pregnancy

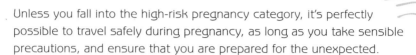

Unless you fall into the high-risk pregnancy category, it's perfectly possible to travel safely during pregnancy, as long as you take sensible precautions, and ensure that you are prepared for the unexpected.

- ○ **Before planning your trip**, consult your doctor to discuss any potential risks particular to your pregnancy
- ○ **Avoid travelling to parts of the world** where there is a high risk of disease
- ○ **Avoid live vaccines**, such as chicken pox, measles, mumps, and rubella, as these are not usually recommended in pregnancy
- ○ **Remember that oral vaccines** to protect against yellow fever, typhoid, polio, and anthrax are contraindicated during pregnancy
- ○ **Tetanus, hepatitis, and flu jabs** are considered to be safe
- ○ **Take with you any regular medication or remedies** – you may not be able to find what you need at your destination, or you may be delayed
- ○ **Check with your airline in advance**: some won't allow you to fly past 35 weeks, and some require a doctor's letter
- ○ **Check your travel-insurance policy** to be sure that pregnancy is covered
- ○ **Arrange for an aisle or bulkhead seat** for extra leg room
- ○ **Wear your seat belt under your belly** and across your lap
- ○ **Reduce the risk of deep-vein thrombosis**, which is more likely during pregnancy, by drinking plenty of fluids, remaining as mobile as you can, and wearing support stockings while flying
- ○ **In developing countries**, only eat fruit you have peeled yourself; avoid leafy greens and salads, which may have been washed in contaminated water
- ○ **Drink bottled water**
- ○ **Travel light** and make sure you can easily pull or carry your luggage
- ○ _____
- ○ _____
- ○ _____

Dealing with sleep problems

Feeling exhausted throughout pregnancy is absolutely normal, but the weight of your baby can make it difficult to sleep and common pregnancy symptoms often occur at night. However, help is at hand.

○ **Get regular exercise**, which encourages healthy, restful sleep

○ **Eat tryptophan-rich foods** before bed (see page 20)

○ **Have a warm (not hot) bath** about 30 minutes before bedtime, and add 8–10 drops of lavender or Roman chamomile oil to encourage sleep

○ **If you suffer from restless legs**, increase your intake of folic acid (see page 18), and, when it strikes, immerse your feet in a bucket of cold water, then return to bed with your feet raised on a pillow

○ **Avoid caffeine and other stimulants**, which discourage sleep

○ **Try the herbal remedies** valerian and passiflora, which are both safe during pregnancy, and can be drunk before bed to encourage relaxation

○ **Try the homeopathic remedies** Passiflora 6C, Coffea cruda 6C, and Nux vomica 6C – these are all good for sleep problems

○ **Take a daytime nap** when you can to ensure you get the sleep you need

○ **Use cushions and pillows** to support your growing bump while you sleep

○ ....

○ ....

○ ....

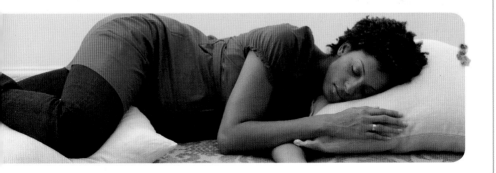

Ideal exercise

Even if you've had a sedentary lifestyle until now, you can safely start an exercise programme during pregnancy – just check with your midwife before you get going. Not only will exercise help you maintain a healthy weight, but it will also promote restful sleep, encourage circulation and elimination, reduce tension, and get your feel-good endorphins flowing.

- **Don't exercise to lose weight** or suddenly become "fit"; instead, exercise at a mild to moderate level
- **Start slowly and build up**: 15–20 minutes at a time, three days a week, is plenty for beginners
- **Never exercise past the point at which you can no longer talk**
- **Swimming** will help keep you fit and supple without putting pressure on your joints
- **Yoga** eases tension, and encourages flexibility and strength

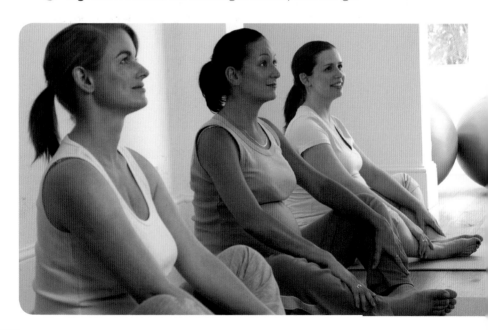

- ○ **Walking** – even gentle – is an easy way to stay fit and experience the benefits of exercise
- ○ **Running and jogging** are fine, if you've done them before – make sure you have good shoes, and don't push yourself too hard; this is great training for chasing your toddler-to-be
- ○ **Cycling** supports your weight, but you can be at risk of falling; instead, try a stationary bike, and start slowly
- ○ **Stair-climbing machines** will raise your heart rate and keep you fit; hold on to the side rails for support
- ○ **Aerobics or aquarobics** classes are fine, but choose one for pregnant women that has been adapted for safety and health
- ○ **Dancing** is very good exercise, and can get your heart pumping; avoid spinning or jumping, though, which may cause a fall
- ○ **Pelvic floor exercises** (Kegel exercises) are not only recommended, but essential; strengthening these muscles can help you through labour and delivery, and minimize bladder leaks and haemorrhoids
- ○ **Always keep yourself well hydrated**, stopping for sips of water as you go

- ○ ....
- ○ ....
- ○ ....

What not to do

Some activities should definitely be avoided, including high-risk sports, horse-back riding, downhill skiing, snowboarding, water-skiing, and scuba diving. Weight-lifting and other exercises that involve standing in one place for longer periods can decrease the flow of blood to your baby. The best advice? Keep moving!

Coping with pregnancy symptoms

Some women sail through pregnancy without any symptoms at all, while others suffer from everything going. The good news is that whatever your ailment, there is help to hand. However, if you are at all worried, talk to your midwife.

Easing morning sickness

- ○ **Symptoms are often worse when you are hungry,** so eat little and often to stabilize your blood-sugar levels

- ○ **Drink plenty of water** – dehydration can make the nausea worse

- ○ **Eat a little first thing in the morning** before you get out of bed

- ○ **Avoid fatty foods and junk foods,** which seem to make symptoms worse

- ○ **Ginger is a traditional remedy for morning sickness**; you can drink ginger tea or ginger ale, or chew crystallized ginger until symptoms pass

- ○ **Take vitamin B6 supplement regularly,** as deficiency appears to be a factor

- ○ **Invest in a motion-sickness wrist band**; strap it on to your wrist so that the plastic button presses against an acupressure point on your inside wrist – these are proven to be very effective in easing nausea and vomiting

- ○ **Get plenty of sleep** and take regular rests – this can make a big difference to the way you feel

- ○ **Try to remember that almost all cases of morning sickness pass** by the end of the first trimester, when your hormones settle down

- ○ **Dry biscuits** seem to help ease nausea for many women

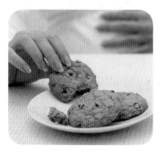

It's safe to feel sick

There is evidence to suggest that women who experience severe nausea are less likely to miscarry, as morning sickness is believed to be caused by high levels of pregnancy hormones, which help to keep the pregnancy safe.

Coping with constipation

○ **Make sure you drink plenty of water**, which helps to keep things moving in your bowels

○ **Fibre is crucially important** – aim for five or six servings of fruit and vegetables a day, preferably with skins, and boost your intake of wholegrains (see page 18)

○ **If you need a little help**, psyllium or ispaghula husk (plantain seeds) are effective unblockers, and safe during pregnancy

○ **Keep up the exercise**, which will help to keep you regular

○ **Try a little reflexology** (see page 36) – massage the base of the heel of your foot, and the arch, pushing your thumb down evenly and deeply; several studies have found that this really works

○ **Massage your abdomen** with a couple of drops of grapefruit or bergamot oil blended with a teaspoon of slightly warmed olive oil – this will help to stimulate bowel movements

Reducing swelling and oedema

○ **Exercise regularly** – this helps to encourage healthy circulation, and disperse the build up of fluid

○ **Drink plenty of fresh water** – this is, without doubt, the best natural diuretic around

○ **Put your feet up regularly** to take the pressure off your circulatory system and direct the blood and fluid to your baby

○ **Reduce your salt intake**, and make sure you are getting enough protein, both of which can discourage fluid retention

○ **Include lots of natural diuretics** in your pregnancy diet, such as asparagus, pumpkin, onions, grapes, beetroot, parsley, green beans, pineapple, and garlic

○ **B vitamins**, found in good levels in wholegrains in particular, can act as a natural, mild diuretic

○ **A good massage** can reduce build up of fluid and also helps to encourage healthy circulation

Relieving heartburn

○ **Eat little and often**, to avoid overfilling your tummy

○ **Eat a slice of fresh pineapple** (not tinned) after every meal; the digestive enzymes it contains work wonders to prevent a build up of acid

○ **Avoid lying down straight after meals**, as this can cause acid to enter the upper digestive tract

○ **Avoid citrus fruits**, or, if you do eat them, make sure you do so along with a little protein, to discourage the build up of acid

○ **Coffee, tea, and fizzy drinks** will make matters worse, so give them a miss

○ **Try not to drink during mealtimes**, as this will increase the volume of your tummy and push acid up into the oesophagus

○ **Avoid fatty and fried foods**, which take longer to digest, giving more time for acid to swish around your digestive system

○ **Slippery elm powder** mixed with water or milk will protect the mucous membranes lining your digestive system, and ease symptoms

○ **The homeopathic remedies** Nat phos or Merc sol (both at 6C) can be taken three times daily, until symptoms start to improve

○ **If all else fails, take an antacid after meals**, or as required – choose calcium carbonate, which is absolutely safe in pregnancy

○ **Remember that heartburn usually ceases the moment you give birth**

Handling headaches

○ **Sniff a little lavender oil**, and rub a few drops diluted in some grapeseed oil into your temples and at the base of your neck – it relaxes and restores

○ **Get a little exercise**, which encourages the pain-killing hormones, endorphins, and improves circulation

○ **Drink plenty of water** – many headaches are caused by dehydration

○ **Apply a cold compress** at the base of your neck

○ **Eat fresh, whole foods** to prevent headaches caused by blood-sugar swings

○ **If you experience** blurring of vision, vomiting, bright lights, or a headache that simply won't go away, see your doctor immediately

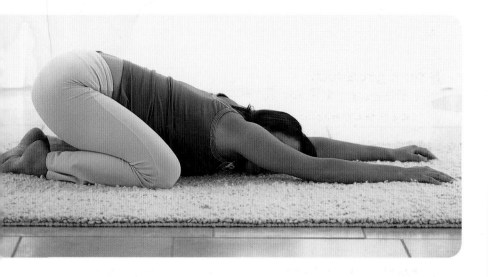

Beating back pain

○ **Shift your position** as often as you can, to avoid putting strain on any one part of your body

○ **Put a footstool** (or even a pile of books) under your feet to reduce the pressure on your back when sitting

○ **When lying down**, raise your feet with some pillows

○ **Try relaxation exercises**, such as clenching and relaxing every part of your body in order, from top to toe

○ **Yoga and other stretching exercise** will help loosen areas of tension and muscle spasm

○ **Exercise encourages circulation**, which disperses areas of congestion that cause pain; it also encourages the "feel-good" hormones to flow

○ **Ask your partner to massage** the painful area with a few drops of lavender oil in a little warm grapeseed oil, to encourage healing and relief

○ **Try placing an ice pack on your back for a few minutes**, several times a day, to reduce inflammation

○ _____

○ _____

○ _____

When to see your doctor

If pregnancy symptoms fail to clear, or if they become debilitating, it is important to get them checked out. As a precaution, always see your doctor if you experience any of the following:

○ **A negative pregnancy test that follows a positive one** – this could indicate hormone problems or ectopic pregnancy

○ **Anxiety or confusion**, perhaps with a racing heart or rapid breathing

○ **Heavy bleeding** or passing clots of pink, grey, or red material

○ **Painful cramping**, particularly if accompanied by bleeding

○ **Any illness that lasts for longer than 48 hours**, such as vomiting, diarrhoea, and even colds or flu

○ **A high temperature**

○ **Extreme headaches**

○ **The baby stops moving**

○ **Sudden swelling of your face or hands**

○ **Vision problems**

○ **A sudden loss of pregnancy symptoms**, such as morning sickness

○ **Severe abdominal pain** and tenderness

○ **Pain during urination**

○ **Difficulty breathing or chest pain**

○ **Extremely itchy skin** that won't respond to soothing creams

○ ────────────────────────────────

○ ────────────────────────────────

When to act
As your pregnancy progresses you will become more attuned to your body, and familiar with the usual aches, pains, and other discomforts. However, if you experience sudden, extreme symptoms of any nature, call an ambulance.

What to ask your doctor or midwife

Many women feel embarrassed about bombarding doctors and midwives with questions, but rest assured that they will always be happy to answer even the most obvious queries, and to take the time to reassure you. Here are some ideas to help you get to the bottom of things.

- ○ **Is everything going OK** with my pregnancy?
- ○ **What can I do to help my baby grow healthily** and stay fit and well myself?
- ○ **Are my symptoms normal?**
- ○ **What analgesics and other medications are safe** during pregnancy?
- ○ **I've had some spotting** – will my baby be OK?
- ○ **What do the results of my tests and screening mean?**
- ○ **Is it safe to have a massage during pregnancy?**
- ○ **Is it OK to dye my hair during pregnancy?**
- ○ **Which antenatal classes would you recommend?**
- ○ **How can I monitor my baby's heartbeat?**
- ○ **Where can I have my baby?**
- ○ **Can I have a home birth or water birth?**
- ○ **What can I do to get labour going?**
- ○ **How can I tell the difference between real contractions and Braxton Hicks?**
- ○ **Who should I call when I go into labour?**
- ○ **How long should I stay at home** before I go to the hospital?
- ○ **Will I have the same midwife** for my entire labour?
- ○ **Can I say no to interventions during labour,** and if so, which ones?
- ○ **Can I have an elective Caesarean section?**
- ○ **Where can I find a breastfeeding counsellor?**
- ○ ....
- ○ ....

Natural therapies and remedies

Many women are understandably reluctant to take conventional medication during pregnancy, choosing more natural alternatives instead. There are a huge number of therapies and remedies that are safe during pregnancy, which will also encourage overall health and wellbeing. Always make sure your practitioner knows you are pregnant.

The best natural therapies

○ **Reflexology**: applies pressure to reflexes on hands or feet to encourage relaxation, increase circulation, and stimulate healing; it can help with pain relief during labour, and a host of pregnancy-related symptoms

○ **Aromatherapy**: uses essential oils to treat and balance your body and mind; it can help to ease a number of pregnancy symptoms, and uplift or relax as necessary – some oils are contraindicated in pregnancy

○ **Homeopathy**: uses heavily diluted substances that work on your body's energy field to encourage healing on all levels; it is gentle, safe, and excellent for treating both emotional and physical symptoms

○ **Herbalism**: uses herbs in a variety of forms, such as teas, compresses, tinctures, and capsules, to ease pregnancy symptoms, and encourage balance; always check the label or see a registered herbalist for advice

○ **Acupuncture**: uses small, thin needles to balance energy in the body, which runs through pathways known as meridians; plenty of research shows that it is effective in a wide range of pregnancy symptoms

○ **Flower essences**: dilute extracts of various flowers and plants are used to balance negative emotions that can be the cause of illness; excellent for shock, anxiety, fear, depression, exhaustion, and coping with change

○ **Osteopathy and chiropractic**: hands-on manipulative therapies that can ease any symptoms with a structural root, such as back pain, headaches, circulation problems, and even heartburn

○ **Massage**: the perfect therapy for pregnancy – it encourages healthy circulation and the removal of waste products, relaxes and restores, helps to disperse oedema, and eases any tension

The best natural remedies

- **Raspberry leaf tea** helps to tone the uterus and reduce the duration of labour; it is safe after the 30th week of pregnancy, and during breastfeeding it helps your womb to snap back into shape

- **The herb yellow dock** is rich in iron, and provides an excellent way to address anaemia – take as a tea or in tincture form

- **Witch hazel and/or lemon juice** can be applied neat to haemorrhoids (piles), to reduce swelling and bleeding, and calendula cream will encourage healing and relieve itching

- **Stellaria cream** will ease itchy skin and encourage healing, and also helps to prevent stretchmarks

- **The homeopathic tissue salt Calc fluor 30C** can be taken three times a day, for a week, to discourage stretchmarks

- **Try the homeopathic remedies Ipecac 30C or Nux vomica 30C** for morning sickness and Hamamelis for painful varicose veins

- **Aromatherapy oils**: try lavender or Roman chamomile for insomnia, tension, or pain; geranium to balance your hormones and uplift; neroli or lemon to soothe, balance, and refresh; and sandalwood to heal, relax, and restore

- **Take Rescue Remedy or Emergency Essence** if you feel anxious or dizzy

- **Massage your big toe firmly to ease headaches** – a DIY reflexology trick

- ....

- ....

- ....

Complementary caution

Complementary therapies can be extremely useful during pregnancy, but only at the hands of a registered, experienced practitioner. "Natural" doesn't always mean "safe", so make sure you know what you are taking and why.

Stimulating your baby

Whether you simply want to spark your baby into reassuring action, change her into a more comfortable position, or start encouraging her to respond to you, there is plenty that you can do to get your baby to move around and to keep her stimulated.

- ○ **Stop and relax** – if you are up and busy all day, your baby will be lulled to sleep by the regular movement
- ○ **Lay down on your side with your bump supported**; this position seems to stimulate your baby to move to accommodate your new position
- ○ **Drink a sweet, icy-cold drink** – this should nudge her into action
- ○ **Talk to your baby** – by the fifth month her hearing is developed and she will hear and respond to your voice
- ○ **Encourage dad to get up close and talk to your baby** – getting to know the voices of mum and dad will come naturally, but she'll be likely to hear much more of mum's, and will be intrigued by dad's voice up-close
- ○ **Read stories or poems aloud** – most children's books have rhythmic and rhyming words, helping your baby understand the ebb and flow of language
- ○ **Singing songs**, such as lullabies, can soothe your baby
- ○ **Music is proven to stimulate babies**, and evidence suggests that a daily dose of Mozart may stimulate your baby's brain and senses; play loud music – this not only wakens her but also stimulates her to move
- ○ **Feel free to play games** – push her little foot or elbow when she moves it outwards, and watch her shift her position; do it over and over again
- ○ **Watch the effect of a strong torch held against your womb**: your baby will respond to the light; this is a good trick to try if you need to keep baby awake during the day to prevent nightly gymnastics sessions
- ○ _____
- ○ _____
- ○ _____

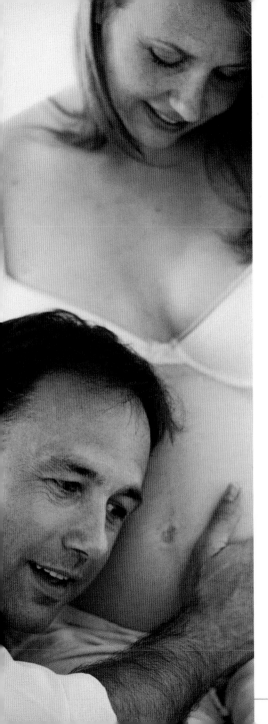

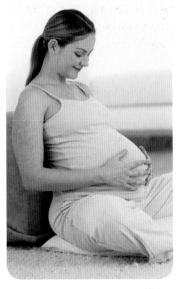

Simple stimulation

Your baby can be stimulated through all sorts of external experiences; in fact, studies have shown that by the 24th week her heart rate increases in response to stroking or patting your abdomen.

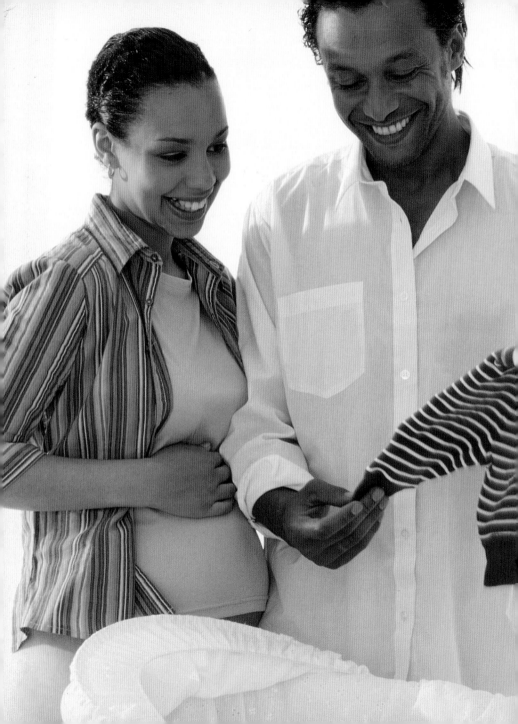

Preparing for baby

Essential first clothes

Although you are likely to receive plenty of clothes for your new baby from well-wishers, it makes sense to have the basics to hand. Try to restrain yourself, though – babies outgrow their clothes very quickly. If you want to invest in an expensive outfit or two, buy them in bigger sizes so that he will get more wear from them.

- **Babies are messy** – you'll need several of each item of clothing to ensure you aren't chained to the washing machine, or hanging on for something to dry in time
- **Similarly, choose uncomplicated outfits** that will open easily for quick (and possibly middle-of-the-night) changes
- **Go for soft, comfortable clothing** that is machine washable and doesn't have fussy (or itchy) seams or tags
- **Remember that your baby will spend the majority of his first weeks sleeping**, so cosy sleepsuits and babygros are your best bet

Aim for:

- **1–2 nighties** – even if your baby is a boy; these are fantastic in the early days for easy changing
- **5–8 babygros** – choose loose-fitting, soft all-in-ones, with poppers, rather than buttons, or zips that can be fiddly and uncomfortable
- **5–8 vests** – short-sleeved are fine, even in winter, and act as an extra layer to insulate your baby; choose cotton, and preferably all-in-ones, which pop shut at the bottom, preventing uncomfortable ruching up
- **1–2 cardigans or jackets** – go for light options, which can be layered, and avoid anything that has to be pulled over your baby's head
- **5–8 pairs of socks or booties** – if your little one is wearing babygros, he won't necessarily need these, but you may want to keep his toes warm if he's having a kick in his vest, or is trying out some of his new wardrobe
- **1 warm coat or snowsuit** – choose a style with a detachable hood, if possible, and an easy zip fastening

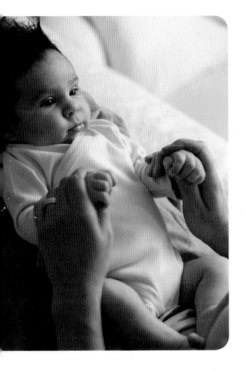

Colour co-ordinates

When shopping for baby outfis, make sure you choose clothes in complementary colours so that individual items can be easily mixed and matched, and if you need to make a quick change, you won't have to replace the whole ensemble.

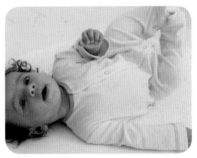

○ **1–2 hats (or bonnets)** – choose one with a wide brim for summer, or something soft that covers the ears for winter

○ **4–5 bibs** – although your baby isn't actually "eating" yet, he'll undoubtedly create some mess with feeds

○ ⸺⸺⸺⸺⸺⸺⸺⸺⸺⸺⸺⸺⸺⸺⸺⸺⸺⸺⸺⸺⸺

○ ⸺⸺⸺⸺⸺⸺⸺⸺⸺⸺⸺⸺⸺⸺⸺⸺⸺⸺⸺⸺⸺

○ ⸺⸺⸺⸺⸺⸺⸺⸺⸺⸺⸺⸺⸺⸺⸺⸺⸺⸺⸺⸺⸺

Which nappies?

Choosing nappies can be a bit of a minefield. The good news is that there is now plenty on offer, and you can make informed choices that are right for you and your family.

○ **Whatever you choose**, remember that babies go through between six and eight nappies a day in the early weeks, and you'll need to be prepared

○ **Don't buy too many of the same size** – babies grow very quickly

○ **Some parents mix and match**, choosing to use disposables while out and about and/or at night, and reusable nappies the rest of the time

Reusable nappies

Pros

○ **Your baby will be wearing soft, natural fibres** next to her skin

○ **They come in a range of colours and styles**

○ **Velcro-closing reusable nappies are now available**

○ **Despite the initial outlay**, they are cheaper in the long run

○ **Cloth nappies produce less waste**, and use fewer raw materials

Cons

○ **Washing produces a lot of waste water**, and uses cleansing agents and chemicals; however, on balance, reusables do less environmental damage than disposables

○ **Washing can be time-consuming**

○ **They can take time to dry**, and using a tumble dryer undermines their environmental advantage

○ **Your baby will need to be changed more often**, as reusables tend to be less absorbent

○ **You will need to purchase accessories** such as liners and overpants

○ **You'll have to carry wet and soiled nappies home** when you are out

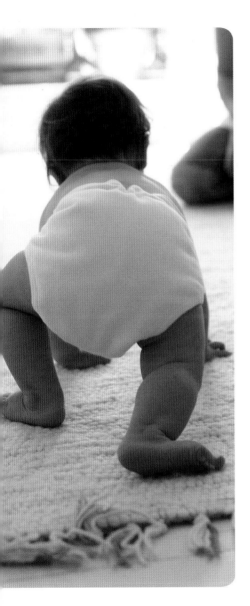

Disposable nappies

Pros

- They are more convenient
- They do not require any additional accessories
- They are super-absorbent, so fewer changes necessary
- They cause fewer cases of nappy rash
- They often fit better, with fewer leaks
- Biodegradable versions made from natural materials are now available

Cons

- They are much more expensive
- They require proper disposal
- They produce high levels of waste, causing a negative environmental impact
- They usually contain man-made chemicals
- _____
- _____
- _____

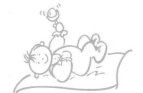

Bathtime essentials

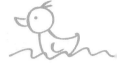

It's easy to get carried away and think you need a truckload of supplies to get your tiny baby fresh and clean; however, you probably need to buy much less than you think.

- ○ **Baby bath** – choose a sturdy plastic model that will not bend and spill its contents when moved; fill using a hose attachment to avoid having to lift the bath in and out of the tub

- ○ **A kitchen or bathroom sink** lined with an old sheet (for comfort) is also effective as a baby bath and is better for your back; or bring your baby into the bath or shower with you

- ○ **Two towels**, preferably hooded to keep your baby's head warm while you use the body of the towel to dry him; you need two because babies often empty their bladders or bowels after a bath, and you may have to start over

- ○ **Baby bath and shampoo** – go for a combined product to save both money and time; organic baby products are your best bet, as they contain no chemicals that could harm your baby or cause irritation to his tender skin

- ○ **A sponge** – natural is best

- ○ **A cotton flannel** – choose one with a pattern to distract your baby during periods when baths are not popular

- ○ **A plastic tumbler or small bucket** – this makes it much easier to rinse hair, and can be used as a distractionary device

- ○ **A non-slip mat** – this is useful if you are bathing him in the big tub

- ○ **A thermometer** – not essential, but if you are concerned that you get the water temperature just right, this can come in handy; otherwise, use your trusty elbow to ensure that water is just warm to the touch

- ○ **A bath seat** – reclining fabric seats with a plastic or metal base are ideal for little ones, particularly if you are using the big tub; a bath "ring" in which babies sit once they are older may also be useful

- ○ ....

- ○ ....

- ○ ....

Keeping clean

It's astonishing how much mess a small baby can create, and it can help to be prepared with a few useful items to protect his clothing and keep him clean between baths.

- **Muslin squares** – these are invaluable, so invest in a whole stack: you can use them to mop up sick, spilt milk, and dribble, and they can be used to protect your clothes when you feed and wind your baby

- **Bibs** – these will protect your baby's clothes during (and shortly after) feeds, and also prevent spilt milk from irritating the skin around his neck; if he's a real drooler, he can wear them all day
    - Choose bibs that are washable, and preferably ones with a wide neck that slip easily over his head; fiddly ties and poppers may prove the undoing of you if you have only one hand free
    - You may wish to purchase disposable bibs for when you are travelling, or out and about
    - Bibs with a towelling face and waterproof backing are particularly good, as they prevent liquid from being absorbed into your baby's clothes

- **A plastic-backed mat** – for playtime, as well as feeding. If, like most babies, yours has a tendency to explosive elimination, you'll most definitely want to invest in one of these; disposable mats are also available

- **Keep a supply of thin flannels** – these can be dampened and used to clean all of your baby's little crevices

- **A pot of cotton balls** – keep these near the feeding station as they can be useful for mopping little noses and eyes

- **Wet wipes** – you'll need these wherever you are, in or out of the house, so stock up; go for natural, organic wipes, which will be less likely to irritate your baby's skin

- _____
- _____
- _____

Soothers and comfort items

You may want to think ahead about whether you are happy to use comfort toys, blankets, and even soothers. These can provide an easy, invaluable way to soothe a fractious or sleepless baby, and may even help to reduce separation anxiety later on. Below are some things to take into account.

Soothers (dummies)

○ **These are particularly effective**, as they allow your child to suckle, which is an instinctive and calming activity

○ **Some research suggests** that babies who go to sleep with dummies have a reduced risk of cot death

○ **Prolonged use of dummies** and thumb-sucking for long periods can affect your baby's speech development, and the alignment of her teeth so limit their use

○ **Choose "orthodontic" dummies**, which are designed to have less impact on your baby's growing teeth

○ **Experiment with a few brands and shapes** to see what your baby likes best, and make sure you choose the size appropriate to her age

○ **When you've got a dummy that works**, buy several, and keep them in a plastic bag to keep them clean

○ **Remember that dummies** will need to be sterilized regularly

Comfort items

○ **Choose a washable soft toy or blanket** and always use it to settle your little one to sleep, and comfort her when she is distressed – it will soon become something she uses to soothe herself when you are not around

○ **Studies have found that comforters help children adapt better** to stressful situations (such as beginning childcare, or moving house), and to cope better when they are anxious or afraid

○ **When your baby becomes attached to a particular item**, purchase at least one duplicate immediately – this can be used while the original is in the wash, or in the event that you lose or misplace the original

○ **To help make an item more attractive to your baby**, you can spray it with a little of your usual cologne

○ **Comfort items become wonderful transitional objects** when your baby is separated from you (see page 185)

○ **If you aren't keen** on your little one developing an attachment to an object, read her the same story or sing her the same song when you are settling her – this will soon become familiar and therefore a useful tool for soothing

○ ....

○ ....

○ ....

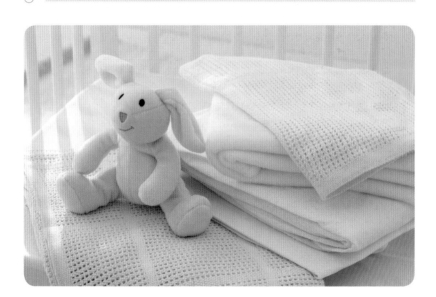

Transporting your baby

There are plenty of products on the market for getting your baby from A to B, and some are extortionately expensive. Remember that most things your baby needs for getting around will need to be replaced in a few short months as he outgrows them, so go for functional and safe, rather than top of the range.

Car seats

○ **Strict laws are now in place** that govern which type of car seat you must use for a particular age and size of child

○ **You may wish to consider a travel system for your baby**, which allows you to transfer him from car to pram/pushchair base without removing him from his seat – your car seat will be part of the package

○ **Babies up to about 10kg (22lb)** – or around six and nine months – will need a rear-facing seat

○ **Some car seats** are designed for only the first six to nine months; others can be adapted to face forward and carry babies up to about 13kg (29lb)

○ **Always ensure that your car seat meets the latest safety standards**, and has a British or European kitemark: ECE R44.03 or R44.04

○ **Look for seats with removable, washable covers**

○ **Choose a car seat with an easy-to-fasten belt**

○ **A new child restraint system called ISOFIX** is being introduced; ISOFIX points are fixed connectors in a car's structure into which an ISOFIX child seat can simply be plugged

○ **Experts recommend that you do not use a secondhand car seat**; however, if it has all of its original parts and labels, fits your car, has never been in a crash, and is less than six years old, a secondhand one should be OK

Pushchairs

○ **Speciality pushchairs**, such as joggers and umbrella types, are popular, but the latter is really only appropriate for short trips, and definitely only once your baby is six months of age

○ **Look for a pram that converts to a pushchair** when your baby is old enough to sit

○ **Look for a pushchair or pram that can face you or outwards**, with easy access to adjust and comfort your baby

○ **Make sure it fits in the family car when folded**, and is light enough to carry

○ **Choose one that is easy to fold** – holding a baby in one arm and trying to collapse a pushchair can be tricky

○ **Consider the terrain you'll be treading** – if you are a country mum, you may need something that can cope with rougher surfaces

○ **Make sure your pushchair is designed to fit through standard doorways**

○ **Check that it has enough storage room for your needs**

○ **Test-drive your pushchair before you buy**

○ **Good suspension and large wheels** will give baby a more comfortable ride

○ **Check out which accessories are included** – some come with covers for rain or cold conditions, change bags, parasols, and even toys

Slings

○ **These are great for hands-free activities**, and for getting out and about without a big piece of equipment; you may also find a sling useful in the house, to keep your baby close while you get on with chores

○ **Make sure your partner comes along** to try out the sling

○ **If you plan to have several wearers**, choose a wrap-style carrier – this is usually one-size-fits-all

○ **If you have back or shoulder problems**, or plan to use the sling a lot, choose one with wide shoulder straps and padding

○ **Chest slings are better for new babies**; you can graduate to one that fits on your back when your baby is a little older

○ **Look for brands and styles that open easily for changing**

○ **Look for a sling that will allow your baby to face inwards or outwards**

○ _____

○ _____

Breast- and bottle-feeding

It goes without saying that you are unlikely to need much more than a comfortable place to sit if you are breastfeeding; however, you may find there are a few items that make the process easier. Bottle-feeders need very specific equipment, which must be kept sterile at all times.

Breastfeeding equipment

○ **3–4 good-quality nursing bras**, professionally fitted, if possible; fastenings should be easy to open with one hand

○ **Breast pads** to deal with leaking breasts

○ **Breast shells** (optional) to catch drips and keep your nipples dry

○ **A breast shield**, for sore nipples

○ **Nipple cream** to relieve sore, cracked nipples – choose one that does not contain peanut oil, which is linked with allergies in children, and that can be ingested safely by your baby; organic is best

If you intend to express, you'll also need:

○ **A pump** (hand-held electric, battery-operated, or manual); electric pumps can often be hired

○ **2–4 feeding bottles** to store your expressed milk

○ **Suitable teats** (see opposite)

○ **Sterilizing equipment** and a brush to clean the pump, bottles, and teats

○ **Specialized plastic bags** or bottles for freezing your milk

○ **A V-shaped feeding pillow** can make the experience more comfortable

Express technique

Most women find it easier to express milk in a quiet, relaxing place. Others find they need to be near their babies for the let-down reflex to kick in. You could try expressing from one breast, while feeding your baby from the other – although this may require supreme juggling skills and manual dexterity.

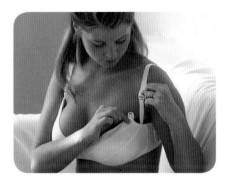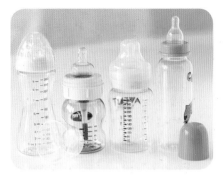

Bottle-feeding equipment

○ **6–8 bottles** – smaller bottles are more suitable for newborns and babies who do not consume much milk at a sitting; you can progress to bigger bottles as your baby grows and requires larger quantities

○ **6–8 caps and teats** – these should be slow-flowing for new babies; silicone teats are more durable, whereas latex teats are closer to the feeling of a nipple – choose from a traditional bell shape or an "orthodontic" teat, which manufacturers claim resembles a nipple

○ **Sterilizing equipment**: choose from steaming, boiling, using sterilizing solution, or microwaving; you can also sterilize bottles in a dishwasher that reaches a high temperature

○ **A nylon bottle brush**

○ **A kettle** – you'll need a regular source of boiled water available, sometimes almost instantly

○ **A designated measuring jug, spoon, and knife**

○ ....

○ ....

○ ....

Bottle choices

There are a variety of different bottles available, including anti-colic and disposable bottles, and even some that self-sterilize; investigate the options and choose the one that is best for your baby and your lifestyle.

Your baby's nursery

This is where the fun starts! Although the expense of nursery equipment can be daunting, most parents enjoy the process of decorating. There are plenty of ways to get the baby equipment you need on a budget, and also lots of things to bear in mind to ensure that the décor is safe for your new baby.

Nursery equipment

○ **A Moses basket, crib, or cradle** (optional) – many babies sleep better in small confines in the early days, but these are soon outgrown

○ **A full-sized cot, with a new mattress** (see opposite)

○ **Bedding**: 3 mattress protectors, 3 fitted sheets, 3 top sheets, 2–3 blankets, cot bumpers; duvets are not suitable for very young babies as they tend to be too heavy and pose a risk of suffocation

○ **Changing area** – a table is not essential as any hard surface at hip height will work, including the top of your baby's chest of drawers or your baby's cot; in fact, the safest place to change your baby is on the floor

○ **Changing mat** – go for one that is easily washed

○ **Baby monitor**

○ **Basic toiletries**

○ **Newborn nappies** (see pages 44–45)

○ **Mobile** over the baby's cot

○ **Music box** to play soothing tunes

○ **Soft rug** or mat made of natural fibres, for tummy and playtime

○ **Bouncy chair**, which can be moved from room to room

○ **Night light**

○ **Black-out blind** – this is a good investment to ensure that your baby is not disturbed when it gets light in the morning or during nap times

○ **Comfortable chair** for feeding or night-time comforting

○ **Chest of drawers** for storage (some cots have built-in storage)

○ **Nappy pail for resusables, or a bin for disposables** – preferably with a lid

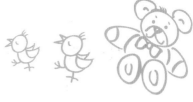

Decorating

○ **Choose a low or zero VOC** (volatile organic compound) paint, which does not contain the unhealthy chemicals contained in traditional paints; or go for natural paints made from water, clay, chalk, plant dyes, and beeswax

○ **Opt for hardwood flooring** paired with a rug made of natural fibres, or choose a low VOC carpet, and clean with a HEPA-filtered vacuum cleaner – carpets harbour dust mites, dirt, and allergens, and emit VOCs into the air

○ **Choose all-wood furniture** with non-toxic finishes; furniture made from particle boards or veneers can release gases such as formaldehyde

○ **Make sure there are no strings, electrical sockets, or electrical cords** near to your baby

○ **Give the ceiling some consideration**: if there is something stencilled or painted on, or hanging from the ceiling, it will fascinate your baby endlessly

Your baby's cot

○ **Choose a frame with a non-toxic finish**, such as beeswax

○ **A cot with adjustable height** will ensure that your baby can use it until she is ready to move into a bed

○ **Choose a drop-side cot**, which will allow lifting access without placing undue strain on your back

○ **Even if your cot is secondhand, buy a new mattress** – look for one with all-organic cotton filling or wool casings, and avoid mattresses that contain the fire-retardant polybrominated diphenyl ethers (PBDEs)

○ **Bedding should be washable**, and preferably 100 per cent organic cotton; it should never contain flame-retardant PBDEs

○ **Teething rails can help prevent damage** to the cot when your baby starts to look for things to chew on

○ _____

○ _____

○ _____

Your baby's medicine cabinet

Putting together a well-stocked medicine cabinet will ensure that you aren't caught out when illness or discomfort strike. Keep everything together in one place, well out of reach of little fingers. You won't need all these items straight away, but it's good to be prepared.

○ **Nappy rash cream** – rashes are inevitable for all babies; brands containing zinc oxide are best for soothing irritated skin and providing a barrier

○ **Petroleum jelly** – this is useful for dry skin, nappy rash, and eczema, and provides a good barrier; if you aren't keen on petroleum products, choose a natural balm that contains beeswax

○ **Teething gel**

○ **Baby paracetamol**, which is good for fevers and pain relief – it's usually only appropriate after two months of age; always read the label

○ **A rehydration solution** – use this on the advice of your healthcare professional in the event of diarrhoea or vomiting

○ **Natural remedies**, including Aconite 30, to offer at the first sign of any illness; Belladonna 30, for high fevers and inflammation; Chamomilla 30 for teething and a baby who will not be put down

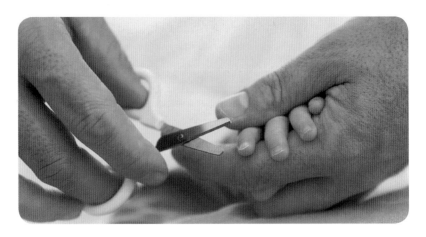

- **Antibacterial cream** for cuts and grazes
- **Baby-safe sunscreen** – preferably organic, and never choose one containing nano particles
- **Medicine syringe or dropper**, to ensure that your baby gets the right dosage, and you can squirt it in gently
- **Nail clippers or scissors**
- **A thermometer** – there are a wide range available (see page 113)
- **Cotton buds** to clean the folds of the outer ear (never put these inside the inner ear canal)
- **Cotton balls** to clear away sleep or crusting from the eyes, and build up on the neck folds
- **Plasters and adhesive bandages** in both baby and child sizes
- **A good first-aid manual** specialized for the treatment of babies and children
- ⎯⎯⎯⎯⎯⎯⎯⎯⎯⎯⎯⎯⎯⎯⎯⎯⎯⎯⎯⎯⎯
- ⎯⎯⎯⎯⎯⎯⎯⎯⎯⎯⎯⎯⎯⎯⎯⎯⎯⎯⎯⎯⎯
- ⎯⎯⎯⎯⎯⎯⎯⎯⎯⎯⎯⎯⎯⎯⎯⎯⎯⎯⎯⎯⎯

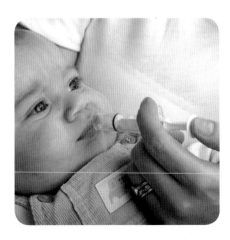
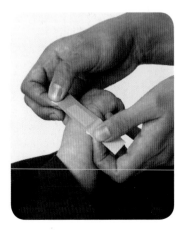

Your nesting instinct

There is nothing like late pregnancy to inspire all sorts of new feelings, including the mysterious "nesting" instinct, which can be alien to women who have previously shown no interest in housework. But go with it! Not only will your home be ship-shape by the time you have your baby in your arms, but you're likely to get your labour started, too.

○ **Get your hospital bags packed** (see pages 68–69) – having this ready will prevent you scrabbling around at the last minute or having the task hanging over your head

○ **Change the beds**, and sort out the linen cupboard – you are bound to have visitors over the first few weeks, and it will help to have everything ready

○ **Do one of those once-in-a-lifetime spring cleans**; you may never feel like it again, and the energy you exert will ensure that you fall into a deep, restful slumber

○ **Consider inviting round a few friends** for a day of spring-cleaning. You'll get it done in a flash, and have some company at the same time; what's more, you can ask someone else to do the heavy lifting and bending

○ **Now's the time to invest in natural cleaning products**, not only to ensure that your house is squeaky clean, but also so that there are no chemicals about to endanger your new baby's health

○ **Open all the windows and air out the house**; get the rugs out on the line, and let the light in

○ **Sort your baby's new clothes into sizes**, so you don't find yourself scrabbling through piles to find something that fits once the baby is here

○ **Give your cupboards a once-over** and check for anything that might be in low supply; chances are you won't get out much in the early days after the birth, so ensure that all the basics are in stock, and in date

○ **Do the same in the bathroom**, and treat yourself to a lovely, soothing organic bubble bath at the same time

○ **Prepare a few freezer meals**: there can be nothing better than having a prepared, healthy meal to hand when your arms are full with your new baby and you lack the energy to get dinner on the table

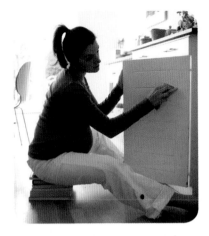
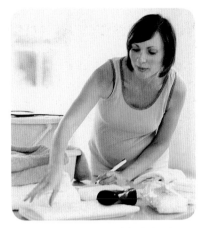

○ **Stock up your fridge** with good postnatal snacks (see page 88)

○ **Make a list of everyone you'd like contacted** after the birth

○ **Prepare your birth announcements** – address and stamp envelopes, or design something that can be sent via the internet, slotting in your new baby's photo and details at the last moment

○ **Produce something creative** – paint your baby's nursery, cross-stitch a little pillow or picture, start a scrapbook, or simply write a letter to your baby to put in a keepsake box

○ **Spend some time finding good online sources** of baby necessities, or create a new "baby" shopping list at your favourite online grocer – when time is tight, all you'll have to do is press a button

○ **Consider investing in a nappy service** if you are thinking about using reusable nappies

○ **Get your finances in order** – pay outstanding bills, and budget for the coming months (see pages 14–15); you won't want reminders causing you stress when you are busy with your baby

○ **And don't forget to make time for yourself** – book yourself in for a manicure, pedicure, or massage; not only will time be tight after your baby arrives, but money may be, too

○ _____

○ _____

○ _____

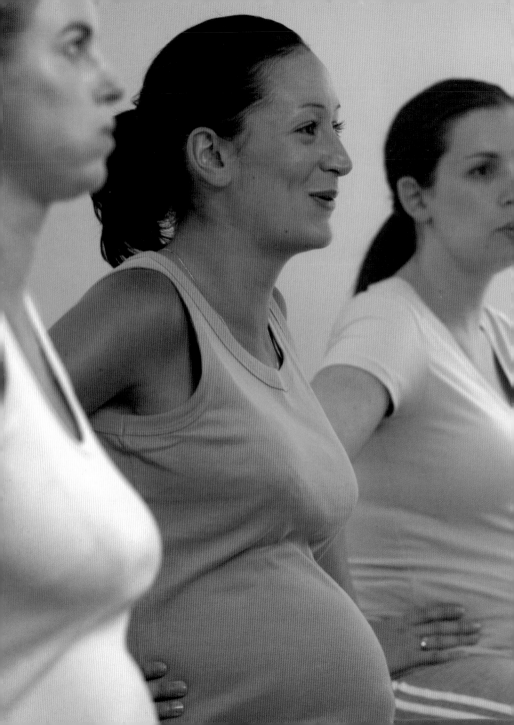

Preparing for the birth

Making your birth choices

Giving birth to your baby is a momentous experience. Below are some of the factors you will need to consider when choosing where you want to give birth to your baby and also when thinking about the type of birth you would prefer to have.

Hospital birth

- **When choosing a hospital**, consider distance from your home – not only for the birth itself, but for any antenatal appointments
- **Visit the hospital in advance** and ask questions (see page 64)
- **Investigate the intervention rates** at the hospitals, especially if you are keen on a natural birth; some hospitals now have midwifery-led units, which aim to support women wanting low-intervention births
- **Find out about hospital policies on things that matter to you**, such as visitors in the labour ward, continuity of midwife care, and breastfeeding
- **Keep your mind open**: you may have your heart set on a home birth, but if a difficult labour means that your baby needs emergency care, you'll want to be in a maternity unit with a paediatrician to hand

Home birth

- **You can often choose a home birth if your pregnancy is uncomplicated** and you are in good health
- **Book a home birth** with your doctor, community midwife, or, if you wish, an independent midwife, who will charge a fee
- **Your midwife will arrive with everything you need** to give birth at home, although you may need to prepare a few items in advance (see page 72)

Domino scheme

- **This stands for "domiciliary, in and out"**, and you will have your midwife attend to you at your home, move with you to hospital for the birth, and then come home with you after the delivery

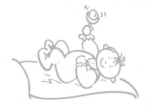

Birth centre

○ **If you are keen on a natural birth**, this may be the choice for you

○ **Most birth centres screen candidates** to ensure a low risk of complications

○ **Birth centres have at least some modern technology** and are usually equipped to deal with emergencies, but you should be prepared to be transferred to hospital in the event of problems arising

○ **Always check out the facilities**, ensure that the midwifes are correctly registered, and that the birth centre is regularly inspected

○ **Be prepared to pay a hefty price** if you choose to have all your antenatal care and the birth itself at a birth centre

Midwives clinic

○ **Most clinics are designed to offer ante- and postnatal care** to complement NHS maternity services, although some will also oversee your labour and birth – once again, this comes at a cost

Types of birth

○ **Vaginal birth**: women who give birth vaginally can breastfeed more easily, do not need a long stay in hospital, and usually heal more quickly

○ **Caesarean section**: surgical removal of your baby, during which the abdomen and uterus are cut open; this may be necessary if you are carrying multiple babies, have a baby in an awkward position, or have some health conditions; Caesareans can also be "elective"

○ **Natural birth**: with little or no conventional medical intervention

○ **Water birth**: using a birthing pool during labour and giving birth in the water; your baby is monitored using a special Doppler device

○ **Hypnobirth**: uses hypnosis to control and cope with pain; you are taught methods of self-hypnosis and controlled breathing before the birth

○ _____

○ _____

What to ask on your hospital visit

As part of the antenatal build up to the delivery of your baby, you may be offered a tour of the hospital, and this is an opportunity well worth taking. Not only will you be able to see first hand where you are likely to be delivering your baby, but you'll have the opportunity to ask questions about issues such as:

- ○ **Parking, shopping, and catering facilities** (and cost)
- ○ **Admissions procedures**
- ○ **What you'll need to bring**; and what you aren't allowed to bring
- ○ **Visiting hours for friends and family**, the number of visitors allowed, and the policy on young children visiting
- ○ **Hiring or arranging a private room**
- ○ **The number of mums per ward**, and whether babies are encouraged to stay with mum
- ○ **How the hospital deals with birth plans**
- ○ **At what point they would decide to induce your baby**
- ○ **The number of babies born, and the intervention and Caesarean rates**
- ○ **Who will be delivering your baby**, and continuity of care
- ○ **Availability of birthing pools or showers**
- ○ **What types of pain relief are on offer**; whether you can bring a complementary therapist or use natural remedies during labour; how long you might wait for an anaesthetist to give you an epidural (see page 76)
- ○ **What type of fetal monitoring is available**
- ○ **What happens to you and your baby after the birth**
- ○ **What support is available for breastfeeding**
- ○ **Ask to see** the special-care baby unit
- ○ **Ask anything else** at all that springs to mind, no matter how minor
- ○ _____
- ○ _____

Choosing an antenatal class

Antenatal classes are an excellent place to meet other prospective parents and form a support network that can remain in place long after the birth. You'll also learn what to expect during labour and the best methods for coping with pain and discomfort before and after the birth.

- **NHS classes** are usually held in a health centre or hospital, and run by health professionals; groups tend to be quite large, but the classes are free
- **Private classes** are usually smaller, but incur a charge
- **Women-only groups** are available, as are classes aimed at specific ethnic groups
- **Active birth classes** (or Yoga birth) are based on using exercise and yoga to strengthen your body in advance of the birth
- **Early pregnancy classes** are designed for women who would like some guidance in the first months
- **Refresher classes** are aimed at women (or parents) who already have children, and offer an opportunity to find out the latest theories and research

- _____
- _____
- _____

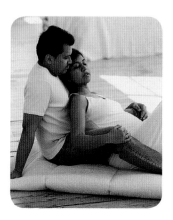

Class considerations

Try to make sure that the class you choose comprises women with roughly the same due dates, as this will help you to establish bonds that will last long after the birth. If you don't have time to attend a course of antenatal classes, which normally run for six to eight weeks, consider attending one-day workshops on topics such as breathing in labour and breastfeeding.

Your birth plan

Your birth plan provides you with an opportunity to focus on the different aspects of your care during labour and your baby's birth. You can make this as detailed as you like; but be prepared to be flexible – very few labours go according to plan, and the most important thing is to have a healthy, happy baby at the end of it all.

Consider and make notes about:

○ **Who you would like to have with you during labour** – and whether you'd be willing for student doctors or midwives to attend

○ **Your preferred environment**: dim lights, music, what you'd like to wear

○ **How active you'd like to be** – walking, doing yoga, using a birthing pool

○ **How you want your baby's heartbeat to be monitored**

○ **Your pain-relief choices**

○ **Whether you want an IV set up**

○ **What intervention is acceptable to you**, and under what conditions

○ **Your views on induction or acceleration of labour**

○ **The position in which you'd like to give birth**

○ **Your views on episiotomies or tearing**

○ **Whether you want to be touching the baby's head as it crowns**

○ **Whether you want your partner to cut the cord**

○ **Your views on taking photographs or videoing the event**

○ **Whether you want to have your baby placed directly on your tummy** before he is cleaned and tested

○ **Whether you want to help wash your baby yourself**

○ **What you would like to do with your placenta**

○ **The length of time you would ideally like to stay in hospital**

○ **If you know you are having a Caesarean**, you can ask to be awake during the procedure, have your partner there, and have the screen lowered to watch your baby's delivery

○ **How you'd like to feed your baby**

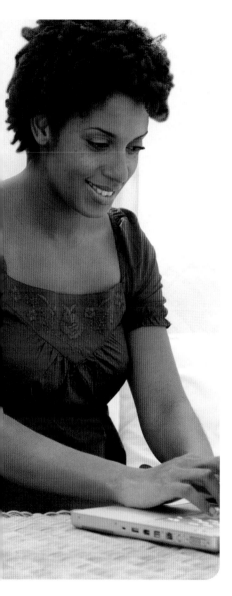

Once your plan is made:

○ **Show it to your midwife and ask her advice** – she'll be able to help you with any information you need, and point you in a new direction if any choices are unrealistic for you

○ **Star or highlight the most important elements**; you may need to change your mind, but if something is important to you, your carers should know

○ **It's also helpful to make a list of things** you would consider in every circumstance, giving your carers options

○ **Make copies of the plan** and give them to your birth partner, your midwife, and the midwife overseeing your birth

○ _____

○ _____

○ _____

○ _____

○ _____

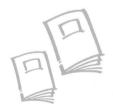

Your hospital bag

It's a good idea to get your hospital bag packed a few weeks before your baby is due, so that you are ready when she is. Always pack a little more than you think you may need in the event that your stay is longer than planned. Remember that your birth partner will look after some of the details (see page 70), so stick to the basics.

- ○ **Your birth plan**
- ○ **Items to help make your environment more personal**, such as candles or your own pillows
- ○ **Dressing gown**, slippers, and socks
- ○ **An old T-shirt or nightie for labour**; 1–2 front-opening, clean nighties or pyjamas for after the birth
- ○ **Lip balm**
- ○ **Snacks and drinks** (if allowed), including bottled water and a drinking straw
- ○ **Toiletries**, makeup, hair brush, toothbrush, and toothpaste
- ○ **Any regular medication** (check with your doctor if you plan to breastfeed)
- ○ **Relaxation materials**: a book or magazines
- ○ **Any pain relief**, such as essential oils, homeopathic remedies, TENS machine, massage oil, flower essences
- ○ **A nursing bra**, breast pads, and nipple cream
- ○ **Maternity pads**
- ○ **Towels and flannels**
- ○ **Old or disposable knickers**
- ○ **Earplugs**, for a noisy ward
- ○ **Your mobile phone** or your address book and change for the phone
- ○ **Something to wear home**
- ○ _____
- ○ _____
- ○ _____

Your baby's hospital bag

You need to take with you to the hospital all the things your baby will need for her first few days. Here is what she will need immediately after the birth, and for her stay in hospital.

- ○ **1–2 nighties** (for boy babies, too), which provide easy access to the nether regions for speedy changes
- ○ **2–3 babygros** – even if your stay in hospital is a short one, babies have a tendency to wet and stain everything with which they come into contact
- ○ **2–3 cotton vests** – preferably all-in-ones with poppers under the crotch
- ○ **1–2 cotton bibs**, for inevitable spills
- ○ **1–2 pairs of socks or booties**
- ○ **1 cardigan** (although hospitals are notoriously hot, and she's unlikely to need much to keep her warm)
- ○ **Scratch mitts** – many babies are born with very long fingernails, and can inadvertently scratch themselves (and you)
- ○ **1 soft hat or bonnet** to help conserve your baby's body heat
- ○ **12–24 nappies** – go for disposables, as you won't have any opportunity to launder reusables
- ○ **1 packet of disposable, organic wipes**
- ○ **1–2 soft baby blankets** – large enough to swaddle your baby, and soft enough to comfort her
- ○ **3–4 muslin squares**, for mopping up and protecting your clothes
- ○ **1 hooded towel for bathing**
- ○ **1 soft, thin flannel**
- ○ _____
- ○ _____
- ○ _____

Your birth partner's checklist

Your birth partner will not only have the honour of being present when your new baby is born, but also some responsibilities as well. Don't feel that you have to organize everything yourself – pass this checklist to your special person, and get him (or her) involved from the outset. Take a step back and delegate. This list is for your partner's eyes only.

In advance

- ○ **Read up on pregnancy and the stages of labour**, so you are prepared
- ○ **Visit the doctor or midwife** with your own list of questions
- ○ **Accompany your partner on her hospital visit**
- ○ **Plan and practise a route to the hospital**
- ○ **Review your partner's birth plan**, and find which points she is prepared to compromise on
- ○ **Attend at least one antenatal class with your partner**, to get to grips with the positions and breathing techniques that will help her through labour
- ○ **Make a list of the drugs or other interventions** that your partner is prepared to consider
- ○ **Pack your bags and prepare** as much as you can at least two weeks before the baby is due
- ○ **Make a list of things you need to add to the bag at the last minute**
- ○ **Review the hospital bag checklist** (see page 68) and other Preparing for the birth checklists

Taking charge

Once the contractions have started in earnest, your partner will likely want and need you to take over; so be prepared to call the hospital if her waters break, or if her contractions are less than 10 minutes apart. Once you arrive at the hospital, brief the midwife on your partner's birth plan, and ask her to show you where to find anything you may need.

Bring along

○ **Any natural remedies,** with a note of when they can and should be used

○ **A bathing suit if your partner is planning a water birth** as she may wish for you to join her in the pool or tub

○ **Some change for phone calls**; not all hospitals will allow the use of a mobile phone; you may also need some change for parking

○ **A list of the people you will need to call as soon as baby is born**

○ **A camera or video recorder,** and your battery charger

○ **A change of clothes** – labour can be messy

○ **Your own toothbrush** and other essential toiletries

○ **Games, such as Scrabble or a deck of cards,** for slower periods

○ **Ambient or meaningful music** to play during labour and birth

○ **Sandwiches and/or other snacks** to keep you and your partner going

○ **A watch or a clock** to time contractions

○ **Your partner's hospital bag**

○ **The baby's hospital bag**

○ **A car seat to take the baby home**

○ _____

○ _____

○ _____

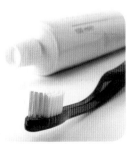
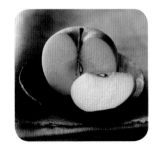
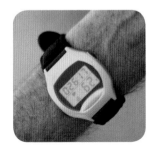

A home birth

Just as you need to prepare your hospital bag well in advance of your due date, it also makes sense to have everything ready for your home birth by the time you are 36 weeks – not every baby is tuned into his EDD. A home birth offers you the chance to create the environment you want, so have fun setting it up. You will need the following:

○ **One or two plastic sheets** to protect your bed, floor, or sofa

○ **Soft coverings**, such as old towels or sheets

○ **Disposable bed mats** (designed for incontinence), which are the perfect size for birthing and for keeping your baby warm

○ **Your birthplan**; you may end up having a different midwife, so it's best to have everything written down

○ **Music or candles** – to create the environment that you want

○ **Any pain relief you've organized**, such as a TENS machine, homoeopathic remedies, or a hypnosis tape

○ **Ice cubes**

○ **A hot water bottle** or a heated pad

○ **Aromatherapy oils** to use in the bath

○ **Light snacks and drinks** to keep you going

○ **If you are planning a water birth**, as many old towels as possible

○ **Rubbish sacks for dirty linen**, and other bits

○ **Kitchen foil** (this is the best way to keep baby warm when he arrives)

○ **A Tupperware or old ice cream container** for the placenta

○ **A clean, front-opening top for after the birth**

○ **A warm blanket to keep you cosy after the birth**

○ **A "just-in-case" box**, which should include items for you and your baby in the event that a trip to the hospital is necessary

○ ....

○ ....

○ ....

A water birth

Water births are becoming increasingly popular, as research shows that they can benefit both mum and baby. If you hire a tub, or use one at a birth centre or hospital, most essential items should be provided. If you are at home, put together the "home birth" checklist opposite; for hospital, pack your hospital bag. You may want to consider:

○ **Making sure that your midwife is experienced with water births**

○ **Ensuring that your baby can be monitored** if you have him in water

○ **Asking about the number of women who have used the pool** in the hospital, and if there have been any problems in the past

○ **Asking about the likelihood of the pool being available** when you need it

○ **The cost, if there is one**

○ **Taking a course with a branch of the Active Birth Centre**, where staff have experience in preparing women for water births

○ **Talking to women who have had a water birth**, to discover what they found useful, and when they got into and out of the pool

○ **If you are hiring a tub**, making sure it is big enough to sit in comfortably and deep enough to reach your armpit

○ **Making sure your floor is strong enough** to support the weight of a full tub with occupants; there should also be room to allow for access from all sides

○ **Making sure your tap adaptor fits the water outlet** you will be using

○ **Adding a cup of sea salt** per tub to prevent your skin from becoming wrinkly and waterlogged

○ **Keeping a good supply of fresh, clean towels** at the ready

○ **Experimenting with positions in advance**; you may wish to use inflatables for support, or a folded towel or rubber mat to protect your knees

○ **Keeping a spray bottle of water and some fresh drinking water** handy; you can become hot and bothered, as well as thirsty, in the warm water

○ ....

○ ....

○ ....

Symptoms of labour

Towards the end of pregnancy many women experience Braxton Hicks (or practice) contractions, which can be easily mistaken for the real thing. Before you find yourself rushing off to hospital, check this list to be sure you've passed the real starting line.

Preparing for the birth

Look out for:

- ○ **A profuse emptying of the bowels**, vomiting, or nausea just before your body swings into action
- ○ **Lower back pain**
- ○ **Strong nesting urges** (when you start ironing the tea towels, it's a sign that something's up)
- ○ **Cramping**, which feels rather like your menstrual period
- ○ **Regular contractions** that become increasingly close together and painful (although don't be surprised if they stop – this is normal, too)
- ○ **In early labour you are usually able to converse between contractions**, and behave normally
- ○ **Losing your mucus plug** – the collection of mucus that plugs the cervix; this can be bloodstained, and is called a "show"
- ○ **Your waters breaking**, which can be a slow drip-drip, or a rush; don't be alarmed by the quantity of water – there's a lot in there
- ○ _____
- ○ _____
- ○ _____

Quick deliveries
While labour can take at least a few hours (and often much more) in most first-timers, some women do experience faster births. If the contractions are coming thick and fast, or you develop the urge to push at any stage, get yourself to hospital, or phone the midwife immediately.

74

Questions about procedures

Not surprisingly, many women and their birth partners are daunted by the experience of labour and childbirth, and unsure about when they should speak up, and what they can ask. The most important thing is that you feel confident about your care. If you have concerns, make them known immediately, and ask *any* questions that enter your mind.

- **Ask exactly what any suggested procedure entails** and how it's done
- **Ask about how painful it will be**, if there are any risks to your baby, and any general side effects
- **Ask about the alternatives**
- **Ask why a particular procedure is being suggested** – and whether it is absolutely necessary
- **Ask if a procedure or intervention is established and traditionally used**, or if it is experimental
- **Ask how a drug or intervention will affect** the progress of your labour, your recovery, and the health of your baby
- **Ask what will happen if your labour is slowed**, or if things do not work according to plan
- **Ask about the pros and cons of a treatment** – these should be spelled out
- **Ask for time to discuss the options with your birth partner**, and for the opportunity to ask more questions – or for a second opinion
- **Ask if you can delay intervention**, and if there is any harm in waiting
- **Ask to be notified if there is anything happening that could affect the health of your baby**, as soon as it happens
- **Ask to be told the cut-off periods for interventions**, so that you can consider them; for example, if you are sure you want an epidural, find out how far in advance do you need to ask

- _____
- _____
- _____

Pain-relief options

There is a huge range of pain-relief options for labour available from both conventional medicine and natural therapies. Many women choose to combine these two disciplines, others wish to go as natural as possible, while the remainder will only consider conventional pain relief. Here is a guide to what your hospital or birth centre should offer.

- **TENS** (transcutaneous electrical nerve stimulation) is used in early labour. It involves attaching pads to your back through which a low voltage electrical current is passed, stimulating your body to produce its own pain-relieving substances. Some women find it invaluable; others find it ineffective

- **Gas and air** (entonox): a pain-relieving mixture of oxygen and nitrous oxide, designed to cause pain relief without undue sleepiness. It works in less than a minute, and can be used throughout the labour and delivery. Although it crosses the placenta, it has no known effect on babies. Some women feel "out of control", nauseous, dry-mouthed, or light-headed

- **Pain-killing injections**: Pethidine tends to be used most often, as well as diamorphine and meptazinol, and they are administered by needle into the muscle of your thigh or bottom. Occasionally, they are used intravenously; sometimes they can be programmed so that you can administer the drug to yourself. Side effects include nausea, vomiting, and drowsiness, and these drugs can affect your baby's breathing and make her sleepy

- **Epidural anaesthesia** involves bathing the nerves that run through your lower back between your uterus and birth canal and your brain with a local anaesthetic. A fine tube is placed in the region of the nerves, and painkiller is injected and topped up as required. Once the tube is in position, you will not be aware of it. In a standard epidural your legs will feel quite heavy; you can get a weaker version, known as a "mobile epidural", which allows you to move a little more. Side effects can include headaches or low blood pressure during and after an epidural, but there are very few other symptoms and your baby should not be affected

- ....

- ....

- ....

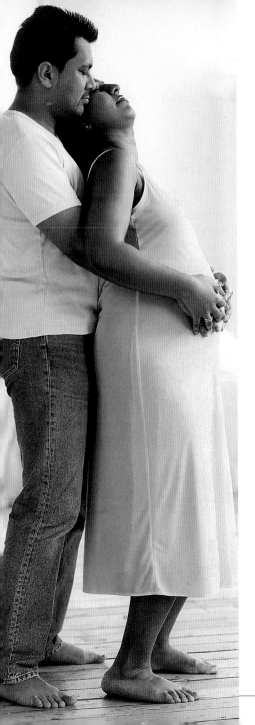

Self-help pain relief

Pain-relief methods that don't involve drugs include massage (by your partner or a friend), relaxation (which you should learn at antenatal classes), breathing exercises (learned at antenatal classes), water (in a bath, shower, or birthing pool), and gentle exercise. These are all effective in the early stages of labour. There are also a variety of natural therapies that many women find effective, including reflexology, aromatherapy, homeopathy, herbalism, acupuncture, and hypnosis. You can arrange for a therapist to create a remedy kit to deal with the various stages of labour, to provide you with advice and treatment in advance, or to accompany you during labour. Always choose a registered, experienced practitioner.

Your gift wish list

More and more parents-to-be are registering gift ideas in advance of the birth, or putting together a "gift wish list" on one or more websites or at department stores. Not only does this ensure that you get exactly what you need, but people will be able to club together to purchase some of the bigger items of baby equipment.

Great ideas for your gift wish list can include:

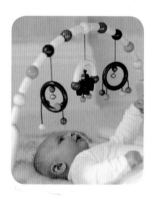

- ○ **Baby monitor**
- ○ **Pushchair and/or car seat**
- ○ **Change table**
- ○ **Music box or mobile**
- ○ **Baby sling**
- ○ **Clothes** (choose various sizes)
- ○ **Activity centre**
- ○ **Bath towels**
- ○ **Changing bag**
- ○ **Voucher for baby massage**
- ○ **Baby CD player** and a selection of soothing and stimulating music
- ○ **Photo session** for the new family

...and not everything has to cost money:

- ○ **A night or two's free babysitting**
- ○ **A meal or two for the freezer**
- ○ **A household tidy-up** or ironing session
- ○ _____
- ○ _____
- ○ _____

Visitors and support

To get through the early days of life with your new baby, it can help enormously to have a good support network set up in advance. But remember that while helpful friends and another pair of hands can be useful, you'll also need some time alone with your partner and baby.

- ○ **A great idea is to set up a rota**, so that you aren't inundated with guests arriving at the same time, all wanting cups of tea
- ○ **Encourage guests to call first** to see when would be a good time to drop by
- ○ **Try to limit the number of guests you have in the early days**, and make sure that they are pre-warned that visits will be short
- ○ **If friends ask to help**, suggest they come round for a few hours in the afternoon perhaps, to help get a meal on the table and hold your baby while you get some much-needed rest
- ○ **Consider putting a list on the fridge**, in bold letters, saying something like: "If you'd like to help …" and listing the things that would be useful
- ○ **Welcome all offers of meals**
- ○ **If you have other children, make sure they don't get lost in the excitement**, or that the stream of visitors doesn't send them off schedule
- ○ **While some thoughtful visitors may remember to bring a small gift for older siblings** some will forget, so you may want to put some treats by for these occasions to alleviate hurt feelings
- ○ **Some families find it easier to organize an open house party**, to get the visiting over and done with; make sure it's on a pot-luck basis, and get in a supply of paper plates
- ○ _____
- ○ _____

Help at hand
Make sure you keep handy the number for your local breastfeeding counsellor and midwife, so that you can ask for advice as you need it.

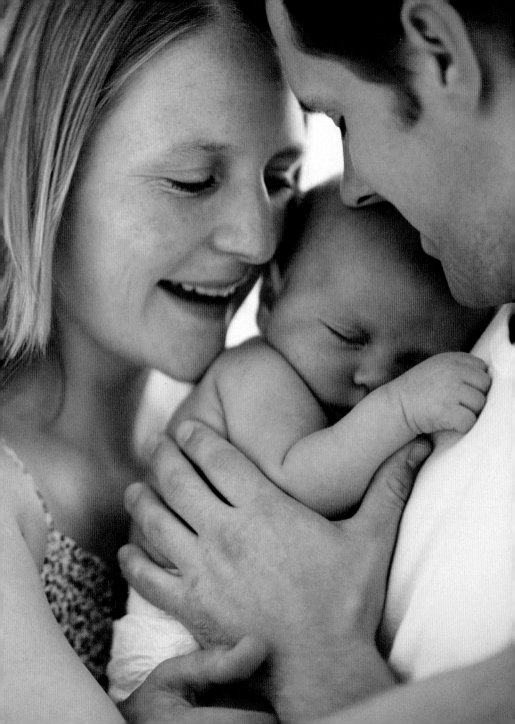

Your new baby: after the birth

Postnatal checks and tests

Your baby will be examined immediately after the birth, and again before you are discharged from the hospital. If you have your baby at home, she'll be checked by a midwife and you may be invited to the maternity unit for a paediatric check. Your health and wellbeing are just as important, and you can also expect regular checks.

Your baby

- ○ **The Apgar test** is performed at one and five minutes after the birth; this rates your baby's skin colour, breathing, heart rate/pulse, movement, and crying/response to stimuli, with a total possible score of 10

- ○ **Your baby will be weighed and measured**, and the circumference of her head will be noted

- ○ **Your baby's mouth will be checked for signs of thrush** and her eyes will be checked for any infection

- ○ **Most newborn babies are routinely offered vitamin K**, either by injection or orally – vitamin K is important for helping blood to clot and a small number of babies (1 in 10,000) suffer from vitamin K deficiency bleeding

- ○ **Babies are now routinely screened in the UK for MCADD**, a rare condition that affects the way the body converts fat into energy

- ○ **Your baby's hearing will be screened** at birth, or very soon after, in hospital, or by your healthcare professional at home

- ○ **Within 48 hours your baby will be given a top-to-toe assessment** to check for any problems – this involves examining her head, ears and eyes, mouth, skin, heart, lungs, genitals, hands and feet, spine, hips, and reflexes

- ○ **Your midwife will regularly check your baby's skin and colour** for signs of jaundice, and ask about her nappies to be sure she is having both wet and dirty nappies regularly

- ○ **Your baby's cord stump will be checked** regularly to ensure it is drying

- ○ **A heel prick blood test** will be carried about before your baby is a week old; this tests for an enzyme deficiency (phenylketonuria), thyroid deficiency, sickle cell disorders, and cystic fibrosis

- ○ **At six to eight weeks**, your baby will be given a full check-up by her GP

You

Straight after the birth

○ **Your midwife will check your uterus** to be sure it's firm, and that there are no retained products of the birth

○ **Bleeding and discharge** will be assessed

○ **Your blood pressure** will be checked

○ **A vaginal examination** may be offered if there is abnormal bleeding, problems with vaginal tears, unusual pain, or if you had an episiotomy

○ **Your blood will be checked** if you were previously anaemic

○ **You'll need to confirm that your bladder and bowel** are functioning well

○ **Your urine** may be tested to be sure your kidneys are working properly, and that there is no infection

○ **Your Caesarean scar or perineum** will be checked to ensure that everything is healing well

○ **Breastfeeding** will be discussed

At six weeks

○ **You'll be given a full check-up**, with all of the above being covered again; bleeding should have stopped, and your uterus should have returned to its normal size by this time

○ **Some questions about your emotional health and mood** will be asked, to ensure that you are not at risk or already suffering from postnatal illness (see page 85)

○ **If you are not immune to rubella** (German measles) and were not given an immunization before you left hospital, you will be offered one now

○ **You may be offered a smear test** at this check-up, and the opportunity to discuss contraception; if you choose to use an IUD, it may be inserted now

○ **The postnatal or six-week check marks** your official discharge from the maternity services, unless you have complications that necessitate further monitoring

○ ....

○ ....

Home health visits

In the UK, there is an excellent system set up to ensure that new mums and their babies are healthy and well after the birth. The number and timing of visits varies in different areas, but you can expect to see your midwife and health visitor regularly in the first weeks after your baby's arrival.

- ○ **Day 2** – a midwife will visit you the day after you return home from hospital, or the day after your baby's birth if you had him at home

- ○ **Every other day** your midwife will visit; your midwife can care for you and your baby until 28 days after the birth if you need help and support; visits can be daily if required

- ○ **Day 7** – your midwife will weigh your baby, and a PKU heel prick test will be carried out (see page 82)

- ○ **Day 10** – your baby will be weighed again (to see if he has regained his birth weight), and his cord stump will be checked

- ○ **10–14 days after the birth** – in most cases your midwife will discharge you and your baby to the care of a health visitor

- ○ **Over the next few weeks** your health visitor will visit as needed; health visitors monitor the growth and development of your baby, and provide you with support on health, breastfeeding, and childcare issues

- ○ **Once a week** – you will be asked to take your baby to your local child health clinic to be weighed

- ○ **6–8 weeks** – your health visitor will make another home visit for a development review; in some cases you will be asked to attend the child health clinic for this check

- ○ **8 months** – another home check-up will take place

- ○ ....

- ○ ....

- ○ ....

Detecting postnatal illness (PNI)

PNI affects about 10–15 per cent of all new mums. The symptoms differ from woman to woman, and it's normal to experience at least some of these after birth. It's important, however, to look out for the following symptoms – be honest with yourself about how you are feeling, and talk to your doctor or health visitor if you are concerned.

- ○ **Lethargy**
- ○ **Tearfulness**
- ○ **Anxiety**
- ○ **Guilt and shame at being unable to be happy**
- ○ **Irritability**
- ○ **Confusion**
- ○ **Disturbed sleep and excessive exhaustion**
- ○ **Difficulties making decisions**
- ○ **Loss of self-esteem**
- ○ **Lack of confidence in your ability as a mother**
- ○ **Loss of libido**
- ○ **Loss of appetite**
- ○ **Difficulty in concentrating**
- ○ **Hostility or indifference to people you normally love**
- ○ **Fear of harming yourself or your baby**
- ○ **Helplessness**
- ○ _____
- ○ _____

Allow others to help

There is no shame in suffering from postnatal illness. Try to take time for yourself and accept any help or support offered with caring for your baby.

Getting enough sleep

Having already experienced difficulty sleeping in the last weeks of pregnancy and then the physically exhausting experience of labour, it can seem daunting to discover that your new baby will offer you little opportunity to rest. But sleep is essential for new mums (and dads), and there are ways to juggle things so that you get what you need.

○ **Sleep when your baby sleeps** – if she's a night owl and keeps you up every night, then go with it until you feel energetic enough to try to adjust her routine

○ **Forget about housework and all other chores** – it's more important that you rest when you can

○ **Try not to feel guilty about spending time watching TV** with your feet propped up while your baby is at your breast, or catching a nap when she dozes off to sleep

○ **Don't panic** – you'll need to make a mind shift and forget about the idea of getting seven or eight hours of uninterrupted sleep in a row; if you accept your sleep is going to be broken, you'll feel calmer and less stressed

○ **Even 10-minute naps** will help to relieve the sleep drought, and recharge your batteries

○ **You may find it hard if you are normally organized and energetic**, but take up all offers of help so that you can rest and sleep

○ **Pay a visit to mum and dad**, or a kindly friend, who will welcome the opportunity to pamper you and spend time with your little one while you rest

Surviving sleeplessness

A UK study found that new mums sleep, on average, only four hours a night, and sometimes less if they are breastfeeding, so it's not surprising you're tired. The most important thing you can do is to avoid panicking. Try not to watch the clock, which will only remind you of how little sleep you are getting. Fall into rhythm with your baby, and remember, once she's established a healthy sleep cycle, you'll quickly be able to catch up on yours.

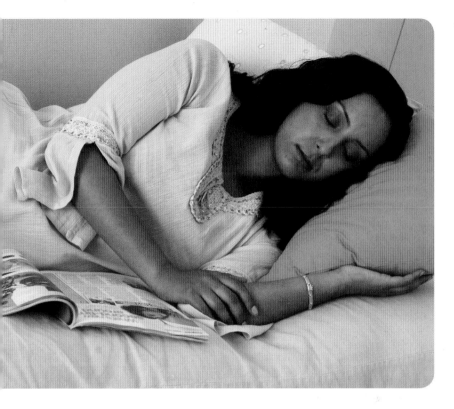

○ **Work out who is the owl and who is the lark**; if your partner loves getting up early, then hand over baby after a feed and go back to sleep; if you don't mind late nights, then take over while your partner goes to bed

○ **Get organized** – if you get yourself into some sort of a routine, you'll know when you can sleep and when you'll have some time for yourself

○ **Finally, pamper yourself a little**: have a long bath scented with relaxing aromatherapy oils (see page 37) then take your book to bed while someone watches baby – you may only read a page or two, but this time to yourself will help you unwind, and you'll drift into a restorative sleep

○ ....

○ ....

○ ....

Best snacks for new mums

Breastfeeding and the physical recovery from labour and delivery can leave you tired and hungry, so it's important to top up your energy levels with healthy snacks throughout the day. The ideas below will encourage a speedy recovery and improved mood.

○ **All of the snacks suggested for pregnancy** (see page 20) are ideal during the postnatal period, and it's a good idea to stock up your fridge and freezer before your baby is due

○ **Try to be sure you are getting some omega 3 oils**, found mainly in fish, nuts, and seeds, in your daily diet; studies have found that these oils are great for enhancing brain function and keeping depression at bay

○ **Eat plenty of good-quality protein** – this is necessary for your body to produce the neurotransmitter serotonin, which has a calming effect; slices of lean meat, scrambled eggs, and beans on toast all make ideal snacks

○ **Make sure snack-time includes plenty of fresh, hydrating drinks** – herbal teas can be iced and drunk with honey and lemon to refresh, while fresh water is even better; fatigue and anxiety are symptoms of dehydration

○ **A little dark chocolate** will give you an energy boost, as well as some iron, without sending your blood sugar spiralling; chocolate is also associated with increased serotonin levels in the brain

○ **When you are preparing meals**, cut up some extra celery, carrots, peppers, and broccoli, and keep them in a little fresh water in the fridge – they're great with hummus or other dips

○ **Throw some fruit and yogurt into the blender** to make a smoothie

○ **Avoid sugary and refined snacks**, such as crisps, sweet biscuits, and cakes – they may satisfy you in the short term, but your blood-sugar levels will soon plummet, leaving you feeling tired and irritable

○ _____

○ _____

○ _____

Quick family food

Time is at a premium when you have a new baby, so it makes sense to create easy, quick, and healthy family dishes that will last a couple of days, and can even be frozen for later meals. Try some of these:

○ **A hearty vegetable soup**, made with a good chicken or vegetable stock, plenty of root vegetables, a handful of savoury herbs, and simmered for a couple of hours, will provide a great meal served with bread and cheese

○ **Place sliced ham, cheese, coriander, and spring onions in a tortilla**, fold in half, lightly fry or grill until melted, and serve with a bowl of soup

○ **Dig out your slow-cooker** – you can drop in some inexpensive cuts of meat or poultry, lots of root vegetables, some wine and stock, and leave it to simmer all day

○ **Make a basic mince**, which can be adapted to make Bolognese sauce, chilli con carne, moussaka, and lasagne; freeze in portion sizes, and defrost when required to create whichever dish you fancy

○ **Roast a large chicken** and use for sandwiches, curry, soup, or salad

○ **Roasted vegetables** with a scattering of herbs or cheese will provide a nutritious and easy meal

○ **Make it easy**: there's no reason why bacon and eggs can't be eaten at dinner time, or try a delicious cheese and veggie omelette for a quick meal

○ ....

○ ....

○ ....

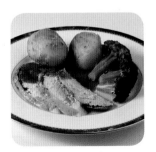 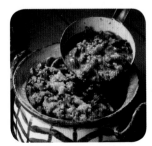 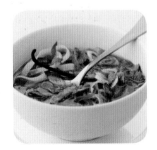

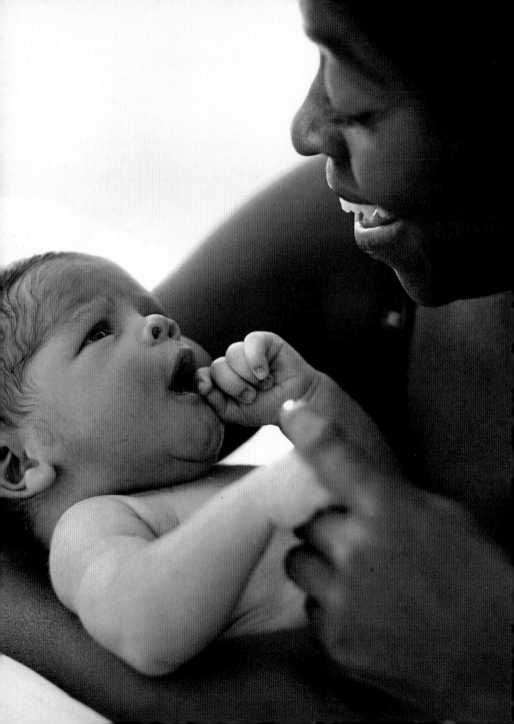

For your records

Developmental checks

Throughout the early years of his life, your baby will have frequent developmental checks with a health visitor or his regular doctor. You can also undertake some checks of your own, to be sure that he is reaching his milestones at roughly the expected time.

By 6–8 weeks your baby:

- ○ **Is smiling and following a moving object with his eyes**
- ○ **Can hear and respond to sounds**
- ○ **Has established some semblance of a sleep routine**
- ○ **Doesn't cry excessively**

By 8–9 months your baby:

- ○ **Can sit without support and has good head control**
- ○ **Is developing hand-eye coordination** – can reach and grasp with each hand
- ○ **Can interact socially**
- ○ **Babbles and responds to speech**

By 18–24 months your baby:

- ○ **Is walking** with a normal symmetrical gait
- ○ **Has normal hand function and coordination**
- ○ **Is beginning to use words with meaning**; may put two words together
- ○ **Can understand a lot of what you are saying**
- ○ **Points to request things** or draw attention to something of interest
- ○ _____
- ○ _____
- ○ _____

Weight and length log

While it is always a good idea to have your baby weighed and measured regularly at your child health clinic and the details noted down in your baby's personal child health record book, you may also wish to weigh and measure your baby on your own, and keep a record of the changes.

Date	Age	Weight	Length

Waking and sleeping log

Use this log on a daily basis to plot when your baby sleeps and wakes. Not only will it help you to work out her rhythm and identify problem times, but it will also help you to establish when you may get a regular break. Photocopy the log in advance if you think you may want to continue recording once this one is full.

Day/time	How long awake	Time baby fell asleep	How baby fell asleep

Day/time	How long awake	Time baby fell asleep	How baby fell asleep

Immunization log

Note down the date of each immunization, and record any symptoms or side effects your baby experiences. You may need this information later as he gets older. The dates at which immunizations are offered can vary between health authorities.

For your records

Age	Date	Vaccine
2 months		5 in 1: tetanus, diphtheria, pertussis (whooping cough), Hib (influenza type B), and polio Pneumococcal
3 months		5 in 1 Meningitis C
4 months		5 in 1 Meningitis C Pneumococcal
12 months		Hib Meningitis C
13 months		MMR (measles, mumps, and rubella) Pneumococcal

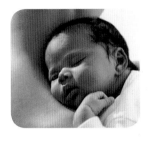

Natural reactions

Many little ones experience reactions to immunizations that can last up to two days. These include a low-grade fever, irritability, drowsiness, and soreness and swelling at the site of the injection. If symptoms persist, see your doctor.

	Vaccination serial number (get this from your doctor)	Side effects

Visitors, gifts, and thank yous

It's amazing how quickly the first few months of your baby's life will pass, and the details do tend to slide into a blur. Keeping a record here of the visitors you've had and the gifts you've received, and ticking the box when you've written a thank you note not only helps to keep you organized, but provides a valuable record of those early days.

Date	Visitors	Gift	Thank you sent

Date	Visitors	Gifts	Thank you sent

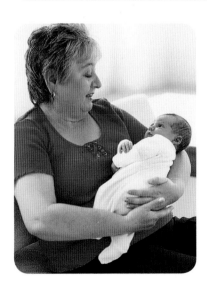

Don't forget...

Make sure you note down any gifts you receive while you are out and about, and those that arrive by post. It's easy to forget things in the early days, when you are tired, rushed, and a little hormonal. You'll also find it's lovely to have a record of your friends' generosity to look back on once everything settles down again.

Notifications

There are a few administrative tasks that need to be undertaken in the first weeks of your baby's life, and it's a good idea to get them done as soon as possible. In particular, organizing his passport means that you are free to travel whenever you like – perhaps to make the most of time off during maternity leave, or to show him off to relatives abroad.

Registering the birth

○ **Your baby's birth must be registered within 42 days** of his birth date

○ **You should contact the register office in your local authority**, and make an appointment; alternatively you can make this appointment at any other register office in the country

○ **If you and/or your partner are not British**, you should also contact the relevant embassy or consul in this country after registering the birth

○ **Either mum or dad can register the baby's birth**, but if you are unmarried then mum must be present

○ **If you are unmarried**, you are not usually obliged to provide the father's details; you can, however, add these at a later date

○ **If you slip up and don't register the birth in time**, you can apply for late registration, provided certain requirements are met

○ **You don't need to bring anything with you** when you register, as the health authority will have made a note of the birth on a central register

○ **You will need to know the time of the birth**, and be sure of the forenames and surname you intend for your baby to use

○ **Check all the details on the register very carefully before you sign it** – it's not easy to make changes at a later date

○ **After registration you will receive a short birth certificate** free of charge, but you'll have to pay for a long birth certificate (full certificate); you will need this in the future

○ **Make sure you pick up form FP58**, which will be required to register your baby at a doctor's surgery (see opposite)

Passports

- ○ **Your baby will need his own passport** if you wish to travel abroad
- ○ **You will need to supply his full birth certificate** (long certificate)
- ○ **If your baby's mother is British**, he will be automatically entitled to a British passport; if mum is married to a British dad, he is also eligible; however, under other circumstances you may need to get permission
- ○ **You may need to supply your own passports** along with his application
- ○ **He will need two identical passport photos**, one of which must be signed on the back by a professional, such as a solicitor or doctor
- ○ **You may be required to get a biometric passport for your baby**, which has new security features, including a chip with the facial biometrics taken from a passport photo
- ○ **It can take several weeks for your baby's passport to arrive**, so make sure you apply in plenty of time before any planned trips abroad

Registering your baby with a medical practice

- ○ **You'll need a completed FP58 form**, obtained from the Registrar of Births, Deaths, and Marriages when your baby's birth is registered
- ○ **Your doctor may automatically register your baby** at the practice you attend if he or she has visited the baby after the birth and you have received your antenatal care through the practice
- ○ ....
- ○ ....

> ### Safe storage
> Purchase a box folder or a folding credenza filing system to keep all your baby's important documents in one place. You can also keep small mementos here as well, according to date. It's a good idea to scan key documents and keep them on your computer, in the event that something important is lost or stolen.

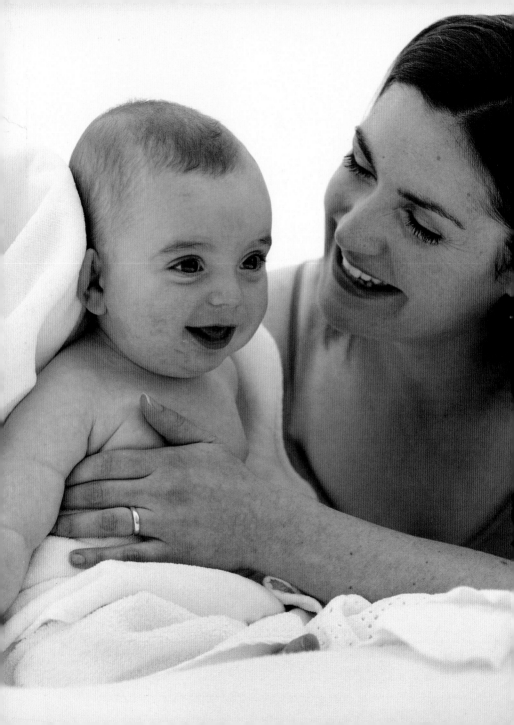

Baby basics

Bathing your baby

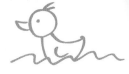

Although it may sound straightforward, bathing a reluctant, slippery baby can be a challenging experience. The best advice is to make bathing a part of your baby's regular routine, and she'll soon get used to it, and even come to enjoy it – as will you. Follow these guidelines:

- ○ **When she's small**, use a clean kitchen or bathroom sink, or a plastic baby bath – this will make her feel confident, and also protect your back
- ○ **Newborns don't need a daily bath** – topping and tailing (see page 106) in between full baths is just fine
- ○ **Stay calm and don't panic if your baby wriggles** – successful bathing takes a little practice
- ○ **Run the water before you put your baby in**, and flush a mixer tap with cold water to ensure that it is not hot to touch, and so that it won't drip hot water on to your baby
- ○ **The water should be no hotter than 49°C (120°F)**
- ○ **Never, ever leave your baby or small child unattended**, even for a second
- ○ **Make sure you are well prepared** – lay out her towel, the flannel, a nappy, clean clothes, and any toiletries in advance, but place them well away from the inevitable splashing
- ○ **Slip your baby into the bath feet first**, and use one hand to support her neck and head, resting them on the palm of your hand or forearm
- ○ **Gently splash or pour plastic cupfuls of warm water** over your baby throughout her bath, to keep her warm
- ○ **Use a thin flannel** to clean her neck and face, behind her ears, her genitals, and between her fingers and toes

Bathing together

There's no reason why you can't take your baby into the bath or shower with you. Most babies love it! Just make sure the water isn't too hot, and you don't use any bath or shower products that may irritate her sensitive skin. Having another pair of hands available to scoop her off you and to dry and dress her afterwards can make the experience even more enjoyable and successful.

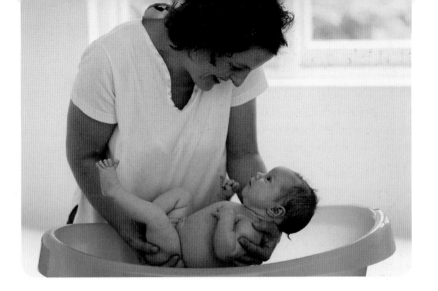

- **Gently turn her towards you** and into the crook of your arm to wash her bottom and back

- **Wash her scalp or any hair she has** with a wet flannel

- **Use cotton balls to clean around her eyes and face,** and if there are any sticky or hardened bits on her face, gently dab at them rather than trying to scrape them off

- **Use a cotton ball to clean around her umbilical cord stump**

- **Rinse your baby,** and then lift her out of the bath with one hand supporting her neck and head, and the other under her bottom; hold one thigh firmly with your thumb and forefinger – wet babies are slippery

- **Lift her straight on to a hooded towel,** and pat her dry immediately; if she has dry skin, you may wish to use a very gentle lotion or oil, although most babies won't need anything extra

- **Get her nappy on as quickly as possible,** making sure you have carefully dried the crevices around her genitals and any little rolls on her legs; be aware that babies often urinate just before you get the nappy fastened

- **It's nice to give your baby a cuddle in a dry towel** before you dress her fully – this will help make the bath experience pleasant and memorable

- **Dress her, swaddle her in a warm blanket,** and enjoy her fresh scent

-

-

Topping and tailing

This is the ideal way to keep your baby clean between baths, and tends to be less traumatizing for bath-shy babies. Small babies do have a habit of making a mess during and after feeds, and from their bottom ends, so a daily wash is essential, particularly for those little crevices around his neck and behind his ears. Here's how to do it:

- ○ **Prepare the essentials**: a flannel, cotton balls, a warm, dry towel, a clean nappy, and clean clothes
- ○ **Fill a sink or basin with warm water**
- ○ **Remove his clothes**, and wrap him tightly in a clean, dry towel so that his arms are firmly by his sides
- ○ **Laying him along your forearm**, with his head in the palm of your hand, hold him over the basin of water, and use the flannel to rinse his scalp and hair; he probably won't need a full hair wash every day
- ○ **Dampen the cotton balls and gently clean his face**, behind his ears, and in the creases of his neck – use a fresh cotton ball for each eye
- ○ **Lay him on a firm surface next to the sink or basin**, unwrap the towel and, using the flannel, gently wash under his arms, across his tummy, around the genital area, down his legs, and between his toes
- ○ **Gently clean around his umbilical cord stump**
- ○ **Turn him over**, supporting his head as you do so, and wash his back, the backs of his legs, and his bottom
- ○ **Return him to his back**, and gently pat him dry with the towel
- ○ **Once again, dry his genital area first** and get that nappy straight on
- ○ **Dress him and wrap him tightly**, ready for a clean-smelling cuddle
- ○ _____
- ○ _____
- ○ _____

Changing your baby

Many mums set up a changing table in the baby's nursery, with nappies, wipes, a bowl for warm water, cotton balls, nappy cream, and nappy sacks or a bin with a firm seal. You may also choose to set up a ministation in another part of the house where you spend time feeding and playing with your baby. Keep a spare set of clothes there, too.

○ **Make sure you always change your baby on a firm surface**, and do not let him go, even for a second

○ **In the early days**, it makes sense to dress your baby in easy-to-open clothing, which can be removed with the minimum of fuss

○ **Remember that many babies dislike having their nappies changed**, so coo, smile, and sing in a reassuring voice throughout to help ease any fears

○ **You may wish to hang a distracting mobile** or toy over the changing area

○ **Many babies prefer being washed with warm water** rather than a cold wipe; make sure you get the water ready before you set him down for changing

○ **Alternatively, keep a sealed packet of wipes on the radiator** so they aren't too cold

○ **Remove your baby's nappy and lay it to one side**

○ **With warm water and a thin flannel, or a cotton ball**, gently clean around his genital area

○ **Apply any nappy or barrier cream**, and fasten the clean nappy in place

○ **Check that his vest and clothing are clean and dry** before putting them back on – leaks are common

○ **Remove the wet or soiled nappy** and place it in the bin; or, if you are using reusables, remove the nappy liner and place it in some water with a drop of detergent to soak

○ **Tip out the water you've used**, and drop any dirty or wet clothing into your baby's laundry basket

○ _____

○ _____

○ _____

Your changing bag

It's a sensible idea to keep your changing bag fully stocked and ready to go. It takes long enough to get a baby ready for an outing, without having to search for changing bag essentials. Try to make a habit of restocking when you return home. Every changing bag will be different, but to help you be prepared for any eventuality, include:

○ **3–5 clean nappies** – if you are using reusables, make sure you have plastic pants and liners, too

○ **2 plastic bags** for wet clothes, and dirty or wet nappies

○ **Wipes**

○ **A flannel**, for emergency all-over washes

○ **Nappy or barrier cream**

○ **1–2 changes of clothes**

○ **1–2 small boxes or tins of ready-made formula**, if you aren't breastfeeding

○ **1–2 clean, sterilized bottles with lids**, if you aren't breastfeeding

○ **1–2 muslin squares**

○ **1–2 bibs**

○ **A spare soother/dummy** – or two; keep these in a clean plastic bag

○ **A spare sweater or coat and hat for your baby**

○ **A small packet of facial tissues**

○ **A blanket** for warmth or for when nursing

○ **Small toys for distraction**

○ **A clean shirt for you** – in the event of a nappy or breast leak

○ **Breastpads**

○ **A bottle of water and snacks for you**

○ ....

○ ....

○ ....

Creating a routine

Caring for your baby to a schedule or on demand is the subject of considerable debate. The decisions you make should be based on your own lifestyle and views, as well as your individual baby's needs. There is also no reason why you can't combine the two. Here are some points to consider:

○ **Forget about routines for the first few weeks** – you need time to bond and get to know each other, and your baby's own routine will slowly assert itself

○ **There is no doubt that babies respond well to routines in time**, as they grow to learn exactly what to expect and when

○ **Setting up a routine can bring a gentle rhythm** to your baby's days

○ **Use a schedule as a guideline**, and don't force it; all babies have fussy days, and there will also be days when you may have appointments or activities that mean you aren't where you should be come nap- or bathtime

○ **You can start by taking a walk at roughly the same time each day** – do the same with play time, reading, singing, and her daily bath

○ **Feeding to a schedule** helps you to know how much your baby is getting, and ensures that she is hungrier at feeds; however, it's crucial to breastfeed on demand to secure a good milk supply, especially in the early days

○ **There is no reason why you can't feed on demand** while also working out a routine – for example, you can offer your baby a feed when you take a break in the mornings to have a cup of tea, or just before she usually has her nap

○ **This doesn't mean you can't feed her at other times**; simply offer feeds at the times that work best for you, and she will eventually feed more during these times, and fall into a habitual pattern of behaviour

○ **Scheduling your baby's nap- and bedtimes**, preceded by a bedtime routine that she learns to associate with sleep, can be useful for poor sleepers

○ **Try bathing, reading a story, and then feeding before bed**; put her down in her bed when you are finished, say goodnight, and leave her – attempt this routine every night, and she will soon begin to see it as a natural event

○ _____

○ _____

Holidays and trips

One of the greatest things about new babies is that they are very portable, and many new parents like to take advantage of maternity and paternity leaves to go a little further afield. Start preparing before you pack by making a list of all the things you need to take, including the items below.

- ○ **Your usual changing bag**, with a fold-up changing mat, and a safe space inside it for your purse and travel documents, so that you need carry only one bag
- ○ **A travel cot**, with your baby's usual bedding
- ○ **Your baby's usual blanket for sleep or swaddling**, for comfort and reassurance if in a new bed
- ○ **A night light** for night-time feeds and nappy changes; a converter if the power supply and outlets at your destination are different
- ○ **A baby sling**: this provides an easy way to transport your baby when out
- ○ **A light, foldable pushchair**, which reclines to ensure that your baby's back is protected, and that he is comfortable; don't forget the rain bonnet
- ○ **A car seat** for trains, buses, planes, cars, and taxis at your destination
- ○ **Nappies** – allow one for each hour you are in transit, plus a few extra for emergencies and delays; you can usually buy more for the rest of your stay at your destination, but pack enough for two days, to be on the safe side

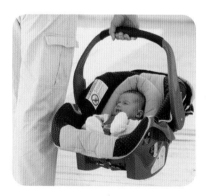
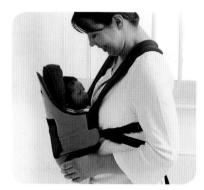

- ○ **Wipes, nappy or barrier cream**, and any other baby toiletries you use
- ○ **Tissues**
- ○ **3–4 spare soothers/dummies**
- ○ **Clothing**: one or two outfits per day; cotton layers are ideal for travelling – socks and cardigans or jackets may be useful, depending on the temperature at your destination
- ○ **Washable or disposable bibs**
- ○ **Plastic bags for dirty nappies, clothes, and bibs**
- ○ **A small bottle of baby's usual laundry detergent**, for emergency washes
- ○ **Sunscreen and a sunhat**
- ○ **2–3 hooded towels**, for bathing and fun in the sun
- ○ **If you are bottle-feeding**, bring along a full supply of your baby's usual formula as many babies react poorly to changes in their formula; don't forget bottles, a bottle brush, teats, and sterilizing equipment
- ○ **If you are breastfeeding** you may wish to take your breast pump and some spare, sterilized bottles
- ○ **Pack an extra shirt** for yourself in your hand luggage, in the event of breast or baby leaks
- ○ **Baby painkillers or remedies**
- ○ **One or two small toys and books** to help you keep your baby entertained
- ○ **A copy of your list** so you can check that everything returns
- ○ ....
- ○ ....
- ○ ....

Clip it on

You may find it useful to take along some elasticated clips to attach extra equipment to your pull-along luggage or the pushchair for days out.

When your baby is ill

Even minor illnesses (see pages 116–119) can be alarming for new parents, but knowing what to look out for will make you much more confident and help you to remain calm when symptoms appear.

Symptoms to look out for include:

○ **Fever**

○ **Unusually long sleeps**

○ **Weak or excessive crying**

○ **Failure to smile when she normally would**

○ **Irritability**

○ **Lack of interest in her usual feeds**

Be prepared

○ **Make sure you know the emergency number** – in particular when you are travelling, as you never know when you may need it

○ **Keep your doctor's phone number by the phone**, and in your mobile phone

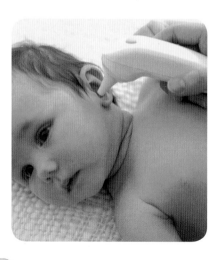
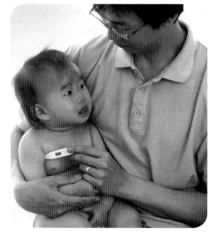

Take your baby's temperature

○ **Be aware that body temperatures** vary throughout the day; as a rule of thumb, 38.9°C (102°F) is considered hot for a baby

○ **Any baby under the age of six months** with a fever should be seen by a doctor; if your baby is older than this, use your judgment

○ **Buy a digital thermometer**: these are fast, accurate, and inexpensive

○ **Rectal thermometers** are most accurate for babies and are quick to use

○ **Underarm thermometers** are comfortable and accurate, but can take up to 10 minutes to give a reading

○ **Oral thermometers** are reliable but, because they take up to two minutes to give a reading, you can end up struggling with a fidgety baby

○ **Ear thermometers** are fast, accurate, and easy to use

○ **Temporal scanner (strip) thermometers** are placed on your baby's forehead and allow you to take her temperature when she is asleep

Check for signs of dehydration

○ **Vomiting and diarrhoea are common causes of dehydration** – watch out for these symptoms: listlessness; sunken eyes; dry eyes, mouth, and lips; pallor; fewer wet nappies; darker urine; and a depressed fontanelle

○ **Breastfed babies** will need increased feeds, and possibly some additional oral rehydration solution (ORS)

○ **Bottle-fed babies** will need ORS with a little formula in between; you may need to continue to offer water and ORS for a few days

And don't forget...

○ **To keep your baby warm, but not overheated** – layers are a good idea

○ **Keep a close eye on her** – a baby's condition can deteriorate quickly

○ **When in doubt, call your doctor** (see page 114)

○ --

○ --

When to see your doctor

No matter what your baby's age, or your level of experience, you should be aware of the point at which to call your baby's doctor – or, in some cases, the emergency services.

Always call your doctor if your baby:

○ **Has a stiff neck**

○ **Persistently vomits**

○ **Is vomiting or has diarrhoea** that last longer than six hours in a small baby, and 24 hours in a baby over three months of age

○ **Has a rash on his skin**, particularly if it appears suddenly

○ **Is under six months old and has any fever**; in babies six months or older, use your judgment and look out for listlessness and failure to take feeds

○ **Has a temperature that is higher than 39.4°C (103°F)**

○ **Has a tender or unusually sensitive or sore-looking belly button or penis**

○ **Is suffering from dehydration** (see page 113)

○ **Fails to have bowel movements**

○ **Has a cold that interferes with feeding**, or with yellow or green discharge

○ **Has a persistent or painful cough**, and always if there is mucus coughed up

○ **Pulls or tugs on his ears**, and cries when feeding

○ **Has discharge from his eyes**

Call an ambulance if your baby:

○ **Is floppy, lethargic, and unresponsive**

○ **Will not wake up**

○ **Has trouble breathing**

○ **Has seizures**

○ ....

○ ....

Baby-proofing your home

Before you know it, your baby will be rolling and crawling, and even young babies can be hurt if there are hazards in your home. Prevent accidents from happening by making your home as safe as possible as soon as possible – even before he is born, if you can.

- ○ **Make sure your baby's cot has a new mattress that fits snugly**, and that the cot and mattress conform to British safety standards
- ○ **Make sure all screws and bolts are secure**, so there is no danger of the cot collapsing, and so your baby won't be scratched if he rolls near them
- ○ **Ensure that there are no strings or electrical cords** hanging anywhere near your baby's bed, changing table, play area, or chair
- ○ **Avoid using pillows, thick bedding, or electrical items** in your baby's cot
- ○ **Keep all lamps and everything else electrical** at least 1 metre (3ft) from your baby's bed
- ○ **Remove a mobile** from the crib once he can reach up and touch it
- ○ **Consider using a safety belt on your baby's change table**
- ○ **Put a carpet or rug** at the base of the change table to cushion any falls
- ○ **Keep small coins, anything sharp, and anything that poses a risk** to your baby (such as choking, strangulation, or injury) out of reach
- ○ **Place all medication, cleaning supplies, alcohol, laundry supplies, and toiletries** in a childlocked cupboard that is out of his reach
- ○ **Place house plants out of reach**
- ○ **Cover electrical outlets** with plastic covers
- ○ **Install safety gates** securely at the top and bottom of stairways
- ○ **Consider getting a fire guard** if your fireplace is regularly in use
- ○ **Place plastic guards** on the corners of coffee tables and other furniture of baby height
- ○ **Secure bookshelves and chests of drawers to the wall** – many babies become avid climbers very early on
- ○ _____
- ○ _____

Coping with common ailments

Almost every baby suffers from one or more common ailment when young, and it's all part of the process of making the immune system stronger and more efficient. Nonetheless, it can be alarming to see your baby ill, and having the tools to ease her discomfort and put her on the road to recovery can make things much easier.

Reducing a fever

Remember that a fever is a positive sign that your baby's immune system is working effectively, raising the body temperature to make it inhospitable to germs and viruses.

○ **Offer plenty of fluids** (see page 113): babies can quickly become dehydrated by intense fevers

○ **Offer paracetamol if your baby is over two month olds** or, if she's younger, ask the doctor if it is appropriate – a medicine syringe makes it easier to administer

○ **Offer the homeopathic remedy Belladonna 30** to bring down a fever – it can be crushed into a powder and dropped on to your baby's tongue

○ **Keep her warm, but make sure she doesn't overheat** – layers of cotton clothing and blankets are best

○ **Check your baby's temperature regularly with a thermometer** (see page 113); seasoned mums may be able to detect a fever by feeling their baby's skin, but this is not always accurate enough

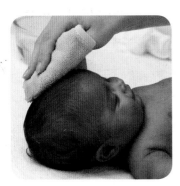

Cooling measures

Sponging your baby with tepid water will help to bring down her fever. Allow the water to evaporate from her skin, rather than drying her, and then dress her in light clothing. If she still feels hot, apply tepid compresses to her forehead, removing them when they absorb some of her body heat.

Croup

The characteristic cough of croup is a definite loud bark or whistle, caused by inflammation of the vocal cords – because the larynx swells and blocks the passage of air, breathing can be difficult, which can panic your baby and you. Croup can be the result of a bacterial or viral infection, or even just a cold.

○ **Raise the head end of your baby's cot** by placing a towel or pillow under the mattress; this should ensure easier breathing

○ **Try steam inhalations** (filling the bathroom with steam is useful) as these will help to open the airways and encourage breathing

○ **Try baby ibuprofen** suspension – this may ease inflammation, and reduce your baby's discomfort

○ **Offer the homeopathic remedy Spongia 30** – this is amazingly effective and can be offered every 20 minutes during an attack, as can Aconite 30; crush the tablets and place a little of the powder on your baby's tongue

○ **Rub a drop of Rescue Remedy or Emergency Essence** behind your baby's ears – this will calm her, which will make breathing easier

○ **Your doctor may prescribe** a course of antibiotics if the infection is bacterial

Vomiting and diarrhoea

These can occur in tandem or on their own. There are a multitude of causes, including gastric reflux, ear infections, coughs and colds (which produce excess mucus), fever, gastroenteritis, and even overfeeding.

○ **Continue offering regular feeds**: bottle-fed babies should be offered plenty of fresh, cool, previously boiled water in a sterilized bottle; you may also want to try a lactose-reduced formula, which can be more easily digested

○ **Offer the homeopathic remedy Arsenicum 30** – this will help when vomiting accompanies diarrhoea; crush a tablet and put a little on your baby's tongue

○ **Massage your baby with a little Roman chamomile oil** – this will help to soothe her and reduce any cramping or discomfort

○ **Scrupulously sterilize** everything with which your baby comes into contact

○ **Your doctor may recommend a fluid replacement** (oral rehydration solution) if your baby is suffering from dehydration (see page 113)

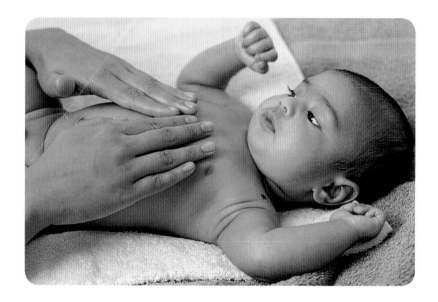

Colic

Colic is characterized by apparently unending frantic crying, usually at around the same time of day or night – your baby will draw his legs up to his abdomen and he will appear to be in severe pain.

○ **Remember, if you are breastfeeding**, your baby may be irritated by something you ate and become temporarily fussy; for example, onions, cauliflower, and broccoli can cause your baby to experience gas

○ **Note symptoms that appear after feeding** and discuss them with your doctor – babies can occasionally be allergic to foods passing through their mother's breast milk, such as cow's milk or eggs, resulting in an upset tummy

○ **Your doctor or pharmacist may suggest anti-spasmodic solutions**, which will reduce discomfort

○ **Offer the homeopathic remedy Chamomilla 30**, which is ideal, particularly if your baby refuses to be put down

○ **Add a drop of lavender or Roman chamomile to a warm bath** to help to ease symptoms and calm a distressed baby

○ **Use the same oils in a gentle massage of the abdominal area** – do this before the evening feed so that your baby is relaxed and calm

○ **Some mums suggest avoiding particular foods**, including very spicy foods, citrus foods, gassy foods (beans, cabbage, onions, etc), and sugar

Colds and coughs

○ **A streaming or congested nose and a cough** can make feeding difficult, so keep your baby slightly upright when offering a feed

○ **Offer the homeopathic remedy Pulsatilla 30** – this is particularly helpful if your baby has a yellow or green discharge

○ **Use a vapourizer in your baby's room**, with a few drops of eucalyptus essential oil to help ease the congestion; alternatively, a few drops in a bowl of water on a radiator will help

○ **Rub a few drops of Rescue Remedy or Emergency Essence** behind your baby's ears to calm him, and help him breathe more easily

○ **Feed little and often**, ensuring he gets enough without becoming distressed

○ **Offer paracetamol** to help ease discomfort and bring down a temperature

Cradle cap

Cradle cap is characterized by a thick, encrusted layer of skin on your baby's scalp; there will be yellow scales, which form in patches – in severe cases cradle cap can last for up to three years.

○ **Massage the scalp with Calendula ointment** to reduce itching and encourage healing

○ **Massage a drop of lavender or lemon oil**, mixed in a light carrier oil, into the scalp before bedtime; rinse gently each morning

○ **Alternatively, massage olive oil into the scalp each evening**, and then gently shampoo away in the morning to nourish and soothe; over-washing will make the condition much worse

○ **Try not to loosen crusts** that have not pulled away on their own as bleeding and infection may result; gently brush away loosened crusts

○ **Your doctor will prescribe** a mild ointment containing an antibiotic and corticosteroid if the skin becomes inflamed or seems infected

○ ....

○ ....

○ ....

Calming nappy rash

Nappy rash results from contact with urine or faeces, which cause the skin to produce less protective oil and therefore provide a less effective barrier to further irritation. Almost all babies suffer from nappy rash at some point, and it can be very uncomfortable. Here are some of the best ways to deal with it.

○ **Change your baby's nappies more frequently**, and allow her to spend time without a nappy on

○ **If you are using reusable nappies**, consider changing to disposables for a short period, as these tend to be better at keeping urine away from your baby's skin

○ **If she continues to wear reusable nappies**, put them through an extra rinse cycle to be sure that there are no traces of detergent

○ **Consider stopping using baby wipes** and return to cleaning her bottom with good old water and cotton wool while her skin is sore – baby wipes can exacerbate nappy rash

○ **Avoid using soap or any other detergents** on the nappy area – rinse carefully with clean water at each nappy change

○ **Zinc oxide** is an excellent barrier cream for the nappy area, and can also encourage healing

○ **Rub a little Calendula** (marigold) ointment on to the cleaned nappy area to soothe and reduce inflammation

○ **Make sure your baby is drinking enough**, to reduce the acidity of her urine

○ **Nappy rash that does not heal** within a week should be seen by a doctor. In very severe cases, your doctor may recommend a mild corticosteroid ointment or cream

○ **If your baby's nappy rash has white patches**, she may have thrush; antifungal ointments may be prescribed

○ _____

○ _____

○ _____

Ease the crying

As your baby becomes more settled – usually between six weeks and three months – her crying will change and you will be able to distinguish different cries indicating different needs. Sometimes she may be hungry, or suffering from colic; she may have a nappy rash, or she may be lonely and just want to be held. Here are some tips:

- ○ **Many babies respond to being held and rocked**, although you may find, frustratingly, that something that worked one day may not work the next

- ○ **Babies often like to have their heads near your chest**, in order to hear your heartbeat

- ○ **Rhythmical sounds**, such as low music or even the sound of the vacuum cleaner, soothe babies

- ○ **If your baby is eased off to sleep by rocking, bring her pram or pushchair inside**, and settle yourself in a position where you can comfortably rock the cradle with a free hand or foot

- ○ **Many babies like to feel securely wrapped**, and you can make her feel more comfortable by swaddling her before settling her down; other babies may feel too constrained by tight covers, and want only a light blanket

- ○ **Some babies need to suck to get to sleep or to settle**, which is why they feed almost constantly when they are upset – if your baby is not hungry, she may find comfort from a dummy or soother

- ○ **You can calm her down by giving her a light massage** with a soothing oil

- ○ **Try not to be anxious** – babies have amazing antennae and will respond to your distress in kind

- ○ **You may find that, if you set up a routine that makes her feel secure** (see page 109), she will calm down and feel more comfortable during the day

- ○ **If crying begins after feeding**, after switching from breastmilk to formula, or after a change in formula, talk to your health visitor or midwife – there may be problems with the formula your baby is taking

- ○ **Try the homeopathic remedy Chamomilla 30** if she seems inconsolable

- ○ _____

- ○ _____

Stimulating your baby

Almost as soon as your baby is born he will respond to stimulation, and enjoy interacting with you. There is plenty of research to suggest that playing with your baby, singing to him, and talking to him can encourage healthy cognitive development and provide the foundation for his budding social skills.

- ○ **Allow your baby to come into contact with** lots of different people, sounds, sights, and other stimuli – what babies see, touch, hear, and smell causes brain connections to be made, especially if the experiences happen in a loving, consistent, predictable manner

- ○ **Talk to your baby constantly**, and give him an early introduction to language; he will be reassured and stimulated by the sound of your voice

- ○ **Take him on "visits"** to different rooms in the house, and outside; show him a bird or a butterfly, or a fast-moving car – everything will be new, and he will be fascinated by the wealth of light, colour, movement, and sound

- ○ **Play music** that your baby seems to enjoy, and use his reactions as a guide to what he likes and what he doesn't

- ○ **Give your baby a massage**; the power of touch is well documented, and it will also stimulate him both emotionally and physically

- ○ **Hold his hand under a warm running tap** and let him run his fingers through the water

- ○ **Sing or read silly rhymes and songs** – this encourages an early appreciation and understanding of language

- ○ **When he's able to hold up his head**, help him to stand up in your lap and bounce a little, which encourages gross motor skills

Meeting milestones

Familiarize yourself with the milestones that your baby should reach in his first year, and plan your games and activities to help him meet them at the appropriate age. This will also help you to make sure that he regularly faces the exciting challenge of doing new things – successfully!

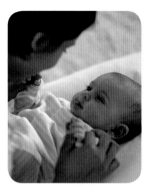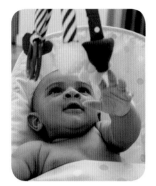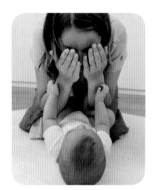

- **Play peek-a-boo** with your hands, or hide your face briefly behind a towel or muslin square

- **Cuddle and hold your baby** – studies show that the more you do this, the more secure and independent he will be when he is older

- **Choose toys that are tactile**, to encourage your baby to become familiar with lots of different physical experiences

- **Jingle keys, shake a box of rice, knock on the table**, and teach your baby a variety of different sounds; he'll soon turn his head to see what's going on

- **Remember that play is crucial** for your baby's social, emotional, physical, and cognitive development

- **If your baby starts to cry during playtime**, switch to calmer activities such as reading from a picture book, quietly singing, or simply feeding – some babies are easily overstimulated

- **Swing a soft toy or ball from the end of a piece of string**, and encourage him to bat or kick at it

- _____

- _____

- _____

Encouraging bonding

Bonding is the intense attachment that develops between parents and their baby. A baby who experiences this attachment fosters a sense of security and positive self-esteem. Here's how it's done.

Bonding with mum

○ **Touch is effectively your baby's first language**, so give her plenty of it; babies respond to the smell and touch of their mothers in particular

○ **If you are breastfeeding**, you are creating the ideal conditions for mother-baby bonding, with your skin against her cheek

○ **If you are bottle-feeding**, hold your baby close to you and let her know that she's safe in your arms; skin-to-skin contact is also recommended

○ **Eye-to-eye contact** provides meaningful communication

○ **Smile at your baby** and exaggerate your facial expressions; even early on she will try to imitate them

○ **Your baby will be familiar with your voice** from her time spent in the womb, and she will feel comforted and close to you when she hears you

Bonding with siblings

○ **Don't worry if this gets off to a faltering start** – the sibling bond is an intense one, and your new baby will be willing to bond with anyone who loves her and meets her needs, even if your other children are less willing

○ **Prepare young children in advance**, explaining that the new baby will need a lot of attention, and probably won't be much fun for a few months

○ **Ask your little one to choose a gift** to give to the new baby, and find something your child really wants as a gift from her new sibling

○ **Ensure that your children feel loved**, and part of the new-baby experience

○ **Involve your children in the care of your new baby**

○ **Allow little ones to bathe together**, and spend time naked – they will enjoy this intimate experience

○ **Cuddle new baby and older children together**, so that they feel they are part of the same unit

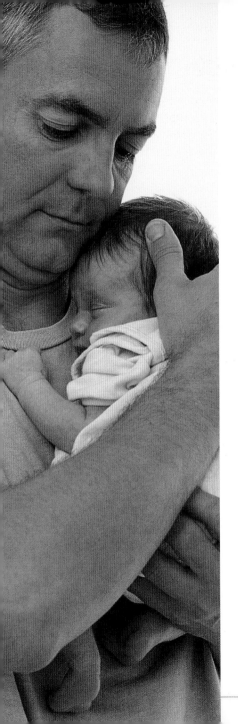

Bonding with dad

○ **Be patient. This normally occurs on a different timetable**, mainly because dads don't have the same early contact with their new baby, and also because baby hasn't spent the last nine months sharing the same space with dad

○ **It's helpful for dads to set up their own regular routines** with their babies, which establish them as "different" from mum, but equally loving and caring

○ **Skin-to-skin contact** can be enormously effective

○ **Dads can read or sing to baby**, and share a bath; mimicking baby's cooing or other vocalizations can establish a rapport

○ **Carrying baby in a front-loading sling** is a good way for baby and dad to bond, as it lets baby feel the different textures of dad's face

○ **If you are bottle-feeding, dad can offer a regular feed each day**; if you are breastfeeding, consider expressing so that he can do an evening feed

○ _____

○ _____

○ _____

○ _____

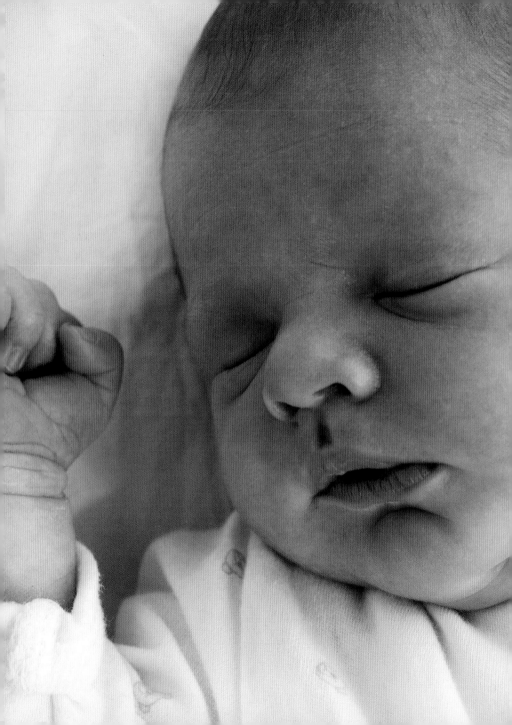

Your baby: 0–3 months

Developmental milestones

All babies develop at different rates, but as long as your little one is reaching her developmental milestones at roughly the appropriate time, you'll have nothing to worry about. Keeping track of her development is not only a source of great pleasure, but also alerts you to any potential problems in plenty of time to set things right.

By three months, your baby will likely be able to:

○ **Grasp items reflexively**

○ **Lift her head**

○ **Suck well** from your breast or bottle

○ **Coordinate her sucking, swallowing, and breathing**

○ **Smile socially**

○ **Stop crying** when she is picked up and held

○ **Use a different cry** when she is tired, hungry, or in pain

○ **Coo when she is spoken to**

○ **Recognize her parents by sight**

○ **Visually track moving objects** or faces from 20–25cm (8–10ins) away

○ **Look in the direction of sounds**

○ **Move her arms and legs** to show interest in the action around her

○ **Bring her hands and fingers to her mouth**

○ **Take some of her body weight on her legs** when standing supported

○ **Have some semblance of a routine**, sleeping less in the daytime and more at night

○ **Control the muscles in her arms and legs** as she starts to grab or kick at toys or people

○ _____

○ _____

○ _____

Best first toys

Your new baby can see only a short distance in front of her face, and she won't see everything in full colour for another few weeks; however, her sense of touch and hearing are very well developed, and she will enjoy experimenting with different sounds and textures. Offer her the following toys in her first few weeks:

○ **A high-contrast mobile** for her cot or basket

○ **A light rattle** – wrist or sock rattles are ideal

○ **Soft toys that crinkle, ring, or rattle when touched**, with a variety of different textures and surfaces to investigate

○ **A soft, washable cuddly toy** – babies often form attachments in the early weeks, which last well into childhood

○ **Musical toys**, particularly those that respond to her gentle kicks or touch

○ **A baby mirror** placed by the cot

○ **Books with pictures or photos** of brightly coloured animals, or faces

○ **Books of nursery rhymes** – your baby will love familiar, repetitive songs and stories… and the sound of your voice

○ **An automated swing** – your baby may enjoy this for her first six months, not only because she'll feel soothed by the feeling of being rocked, but also because it will entertain her as the world goes flashing by

○ ....

○ ....

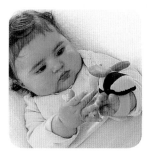 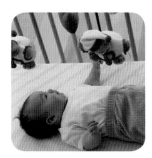 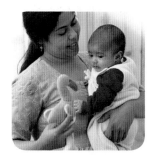

Breastfeeding basics

Although breastfeeding is one of the most natural acts in the world, it can take a lot of practice before you get the hang of it. Both you and your baby may be amateurs, so take your time to become accustomed to different positions, and enjoy the experience.

○ **Experiment with different positions** – some mums like the "cradle hold", while others prefer the "cross-over hold" where they use the opposite arm and hand to hold the baby to the breast they are feeding from

○ **Ask your midwife or breastfeeding counsellor** for advice about the many different breastfeeding positions, and experiment until both you and your baby are comfortable

○ **Regularly alternate breastfeeding holds** – each hold puts pressure on a different part of your nipple and you may find that using different holds is the best way to avoid getting clogged milk ducts

○ **Make sure your baby is facing you**, usually lying on his side, rather than on his back

○ **You might find it easier to put a footrest or low table under your feet**, to offer more support, and prevent having to bend over your baby

○ **Choose a comfortable chair with arm rests**, and use a pillow to support your back and arms

○ **Always bring your baby to your breast**, rather than the other way round

○ **Use your free hand to support your breast** as you feed

○ **Try swaddling your baby** or gently holding his arms by his side to make feeding easier

○ **Alternate the breast you first feed from** – not only will your baby get the hydrating foremilk before moving on to the rich, more nutritious hind milk, but you'll ensure that both breasts are producing plenty of milk

○ **Try to relax before feeding**

○ **Keep a tall glass of water or juice** by your side, to keep you hydrated, which helps you to produce milk

○ **Ensure that your baby latches on correctly** as this is undoubtedly the secret of successful breastfeeding (see opposite)

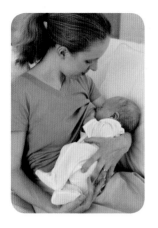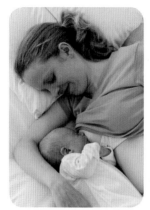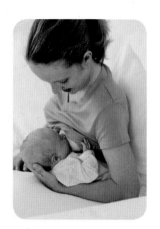

Latching on

○ **To help ensure a good latch,** hold your breast and touch your nipple to your baby's nose; tickling his cheek and lips with the nipple will encourage the "rooting reflex", sending a signal to your baby to open his mouth

○ **Your baby's mouth needs to be open wide,** with his tongue down and forward, and your nipple should be aimed at the roof of his mouth

○ **He should be drawing all of the nipple** and some breast tissue into his mouth, his lower lip will be rolled out, and his chin will be against your breast

○ **When your baby is correctly latched on,** you should hear only a low-pitched swallowing noise – not a sucking or smacking noise – and you should see his jaw moving, a sign that successful feeding is taking place

○ **To remove your child from the breast,** carefully insert your clean little finger into the corner of his mouth – a gentle "pop" means you've broken the suction and you can pull him away

○ _____

○ _____

○ _____

Breastfeeding problems

Even the most seasoned breastfeeder can experience some discomfort and other problems while feeding. Fortunately, there are plenty of tried-and-tested tricks to help ensure breastfeeding is a success.

Engorgement

○ **Check your baby is latched on properly** (see page 131) as this will make sure that all of the breast is emptied of milk and help relieve engorgement

○ **If she struggles to get a grip on an engorged breast**, express some milk before feeding – this will also relieve the feeling of fullness

○ **Continue feeding from the engorged breast**, which will offer some relief

○ **For extreme discomfort, try placing cold, bruised cabbage leaves** in your bra – the enzymes appear to reduce swelling and prevent oversupply of milk; this also works well for mastitis

Mastitis

○ **You may notice hot or red streaks** on your breast, and experience pain and even a high temperature; mastitis can result from severe engorgement, poor latching-on, or blocked milk ducts (see below)

○ **Feed frequently from both breasts**, but especially the affected side

○ **Try the homeopathic remedy Belladonna 30**

○ **Try to express milk** to empty the breast and move the lumps

○ **See your doctor** if your symptoms don't improve in 24 hours

Blocked ducts

○ **The best treatment** for this is regular feeding to get the milk flowing

○ **Massage the breast and hand express milk**, moving the milk down the channels towards the blocked ducts

○ **Place warm compresses** over the affected areas, and ensure your baby has the whole nipple in her mouth at every feed

Sore and chapped nipples

○ **Try to relax** when you are feeding, which will help the milk come

○ **Seek advice from a breastfeeding counsellor** – poor positioning and latch (see pages 130–131) are the main causes of sore nipples

○ **Start feeds on the breast that is the least sore**

○ **Try to avoid pulling her off**, as the suction created by her mouth on your breast can make it more painful (see page 131)

○ **At the end of a feed**, express a little of the rich, fatty milk and rub it over your nipple to encourage healing

○ **Between feeds**, keep your bra and T-shirt off for short periods to allow the air to get to your nipples

○ **Avoid using plastic-backed breast pads**, and change damp pads

○ **There are some good emollient creams** on the market for sore nipples, many of which contain all-natural ingredients, such as lanolin or chamomile

○ **The homeopathic remedies** Chamomilla 30 and Pulsatilla 30 should help

Shortage of milk

○ **Be patient**: it can take some time for your milk supply to become established and for "supply and demand" to kick in

○ **Allow your baby to suckle** frequently, as this will stimulate your body to produce more milk; if necessary, wake your baby to feed, and also express milk between feeds to help stimulate milk supply

○ **Make sure that you are relaxed** when you feed her – if you are tired and anxious it might seem as though there is no milk, or not enough

○ **Take some time to rest**, and even retire to bed with your baby for a day or two, to divert your energy towards making milk

○ **Make sure you are getting enough to eat** – you need plenty of energy to produce milk, and an inadequate diet can certainly affect your milk supply

○ **Drinking fennel tea** throughout the day seems to help some women

○ ....

○ ....

Bottle-feeding basics

Many women can't breastfeed or don't like the idea of it. The good news is that formula milk offers your baby all the essential nutrients he needs and is designed to be as close to breast milk as possible. There are a few things to bear in mind with bottle-feeding:

○ **Carefully follow the manufacturer's instructions** – too much formula powder or liquid can cause your baby to become constipated, or thirsty; too little may mean he isn't getting what he needs in terms of nutrition

○ **Make up feeds with water that has been previously boiled and cooled** – ideally the water should be at a temperature of 70°C (158°F) or hotter as formula is not sterile and this level of heat will kill any bacteria in the powder

○ **Choose a teat that is the right size** for the age of your baby, and experiment a bit to see if he prefers faster or slow-flow teats

○ **To feed your baby**, cradle him in a semi-upright position and support his head; don't feed him lying down – formula can flow into the sinuses or middle ear, causing an infection

○ **To prevent your baby from swallowing air as he sucks**, tilt the bottle so that the formula fills the neck of the bottle and covers the teat

○ **Your newborn will probably take 60–120ml** (2–4oz) per feed during his first few weeks, and he will probably be hungry every two to four hours

○ **Don't encourage your baby to empty the bottle** if he's not interested; and if he's still sucking when the bottle is empty, offer him more

○ **To prevent a tummy full of air**, wind your baby frequently

○ **Sterilize bottles, teats, rings**, and the equipment you use for preparing and cleaning your baby's bottles

○ **Do not use mineral water to make up feeds** as this will upset the balance of nutrients in the formula

○ _____

○ _____

○ _____

Soothing your baby to sleep

If there's one source of despair for new parents, it's trying to get their babies to sleep. New babies can be erratic sleepers, and wakeful just when you need sleep the most. Here's some help for harried parents:

○ **Providing a comfort object**, such as a favourite blanket or cuddly toy, can help

○ **Babies often jerk themselves awake** (a natural reflex) and you can avoid this by swaddling your baby tightly in a blanket at bedtime

○ **Try placing one of your T-shirts near your child's face** – if he wakes and can smell you, he may not feel so frightened

○ **The bedtime routine** is one of the most important routines you can establish – when your baby begins to recognize his own routine, he will relax and feel secure, and he will know what to expect

○ **Some babies appear to be born with their own body clocks**, and you may notice before he is even born that your baby has periods of activity in the nights, which is a sure sign that you have a night owl on your hands

○ **Keep the blinds open while he sleeps in the day** and settle him down for naps at regular intervals

○ **If he falls asleep feeding**, gently wake him and spend some time talking to and playing with him

○ **Keep household activities as noisy** as possible during the day, so he becomes used to the idea that it's normal to be awake during these hours

○ **Put him to bed at a reasonable time**, even if he's not obviously tired; come back if he calls, but don't be tempted to get him back up again

○ **When he wakes in the night**, feed, change, and comfort him, but keep the lights low and talk to him quietly

○ **Wake him in the morning at a reasonable hour** and keep things as routine as possible throughout the day – he'll soon learn that daytime is for fun and night-time is just plain boring and he may as well go to sleep

○ _____

○ _____

○ _____

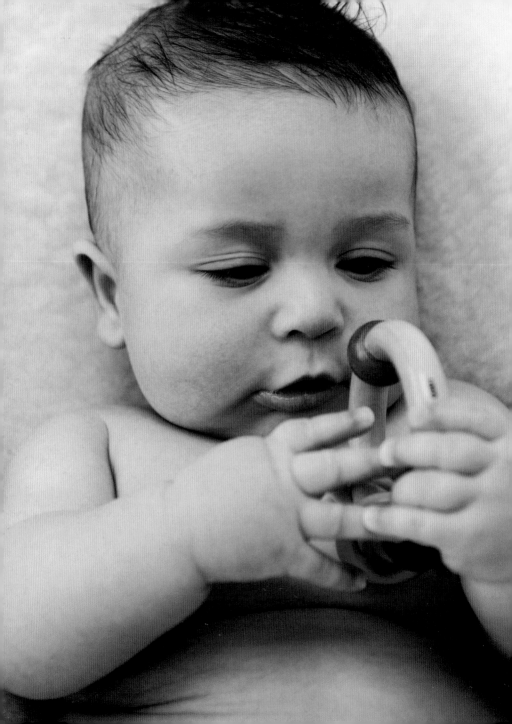

Your baby: 3–6 months

Developmental milestones

You will be astonished by how quickly your helpless new baby becomes a confident, eager explorer, and able to master all sorts of new tricks. There is no need to push her towards achieving her milestones – she'll get there all on her own. You can, however, offer her a little help when she feels frustrated by her inability to get things just right.

By six months, your baby will likely be able to:

○ **Smile frequently**; and she's now starting to laugh

○ **Focus on objects** up to a metre (3ft 3in) away

○ **Follow with her gaze** objects going across, over, and under her

○ **Hold her head up** to look around

○ **Enjoy looking at and playing with her hands and feet**

○ **Push herself up on her hands** when she's on her tummy

○ **Begin to try to roll over** – this often starts when she manages a turn accidentally, and then learns that she can reproduce it with a little effort

○ **Reach and grab things**

○ **Play with both hands together**

○ **Imitate more facial expressions**

○ **Begin using different vowel sounds**

○ **Begin squealing**, as she explores the different pitches of her voice

○ **Become more active** in getting your attention

○ **Begin to sit with support**

○ **Show an interest in food** and feeding herself (although she won't be ready for weaning quite yet – see page 144)

○ **Reach for a toy she's dropped**

○ **Support her weight** when pulled to standing position

○ **Sleep about 14–16 hours per day**, several of which are during the daytime – sleep time is usually spaced out in two or three naps and a solid block of about six hours (sometimes much longer) at night

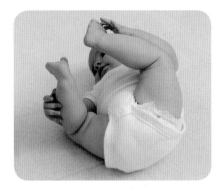

She's now ready for...

○ **Swimming lessons** with mum or dad

○ **A cup**, to experiment with and to learn the basics of sipping and drinking instead of just sucking

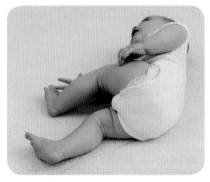

○ **A toothbrush**, and regular cleaning of her gums and emerging teeth

○ **Baby music** or movement classes, aimed at tiny tots

○ **Playtime with friends** – she'll be captivated by other babies and children, and probably want to get them into her mouth somehow, too

○ **A pushchair that allows her to sit more upright**, to see the world around her

○ _____

○ _____

○ _____

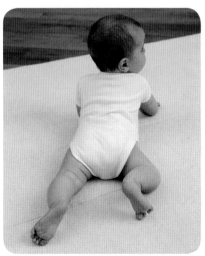

○ _____

○ _____

Best toys and activities

Between three and six months your baby will discover how to use his hands, putting everything he can into his mouth. He'll also be developing a sense of humour, and enjoy playing with you, laughing and smiling when you spend time together.

Best toys

○ **Toys that don't have small bits that come off**, or strings or wires that could hurt your baby

○ **Rattles are the perfect toy for this age**, and although he won't necessarily be able to control his movements, he'll love to make noise – choose one that neatly fits in his little hand

○ **Baby gyms come into their own from three months** – choose one that reacts quickly to your baby's touch or kicks, allowing him to spin, grasp, push, pull, and manipulate the hanging objects

○ **Squeaky, ringing, or crackling toys** respond easily to your baby's grip

○ **Textured fabric toys** help your baby explore different sensations

○ **Board books** with firm lift-the-flaps are excellent for reading together, and are also a good chunky toy for your baby to chew on or gaze at on his own

○ **Blocks with "surprises"** will entertain your baby endlessly; as he examines them he'll be delighted by what's inside and the sound they make

○ **Although he won't quite be ready for stacking toys**, rings that fit on to a central spike are a good idea, particularly if they are resilient enough for chewing, and easy for chubby hands to grasp

○ **Stacking pots** make a satisfying noise when banged together, and your little one will enjoy swiping at towers and knocking them down

○ **Bath toys** that squeak, leak, and float encourage your baby to bat at them and to learn to pour

○ **A music box** that responds to your baby's touch with nursery rhymes or lively music will astound and amuse him when he learns that he can make things happen all by himself

○ **Toys that pop up** when buttons are easily pressed will provide endless entertainment, and he will slowly become more adept at actually hitting the right spots to make the toys jump out

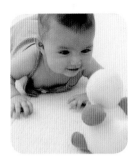
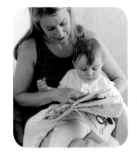
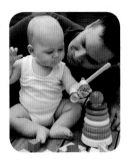

Playtime

○ **This is the perfect age to read** regularly to your baby; he will love sitting on your lap and listening to the sound of your voice as you point out colourful pictures, make animal sounds, and encourage him to lift flaps

○ **Try books with sounds and music that respond** when touched; these will help your baby learn that he can control things himself

○ **Place favourite toys just out of your baby's reach** to encourage him to move towards them – this will also help development of his balance, hand-eye coordination, and gross motor skills

○ **Provide plenty of things for your baby to kick**, including your hands; try to grab his feet as he lifts them, and see him laugh when he hits the target – make plenty of noise in response

○ **Prop your baby up on pillows** so that he has a view of his surroundings, this will also strengthen his neck and back

○ **Place your baby in front of a mirror**: he'll be fascinated by the "other baby", and will often smile at and talk to his new friend

○ **Encourage his cognitive development**, problem-solving ability, and memory by putting a ball under one of his toys or blankets, and encouraging him to find it

○ **Show him how to make things happen by himself** by banging a wooden spoon on a pot, for example

○ **Tickle, cuddle, and play with his arms and legs** as he gets used to new sensations and learns what his body can do

○ **Don't forget tummy time**, which will encourage a strong neck, excite his curiosity, and get him ready for crawling and rolling

○ _____

○ _____

Essential clothing and equipment

As your baby becomes older, her needs will change slightly. You may find she's now ready for "proper clothes" rather than all-in-ones, and she may also be ready for more sophisticated equipment as her world increasingly extends beyond your lap.

To wear

○ **Your baby will still need regular changing**, so be practical and make sure that trousers and other items are easy to put on and remove

○ **Avoid anything too fussy** that will irritate her skin or get in the way of her activities

○ **Poppers and well-padded zips** are easier than buttons

○ **Make sure that any tops and jumpers** have wide necks

○ **Everything should be machine washable**

○ **You might think about choosing a wardrobe in complementary colours**, so that leaks and spills don't mean a whole new outfit is needed

○ **Vests with fasteners** under the crotch will keep your baby warm when T-shirts or dresses ride up

○ **Choose tops that also close down below**, to avoid discomfort

○ **Make sure all of her clothing is loose and comfortable**, and that she isn't too hot – it's better to layer thin items than to give your child bulky, heavy clothing to wear

○ **Babies do not need shoes** until they are confidently walking, but you can keep little feet warm with bootees or simple, soft leather moccasin-type footwear; if they have elasticated tops, they will keep her socks on, too

○ **If she constantly loses her socks**, why not consider a pair of tights – these are a good idea for boys, too

○ **Try to buy most of your socks in the same colour**, so you don't face an endless pile of oddies; and there's nothing wrong with mismatched socks from time to time – just call it your baby's unique sense of style

○ **Make sure that your baby's outdoor wear has a good hood** – babies soon become adept at removing hats… and losing them

Equipment

○ **Teething rings** – many babies start showing signs of teething around four months, so be prepared; avoid teethers that are made of PVC, and look for those that can be refrigerated to provide relief from discomfort

○ **A chair**, which will allow her a wider view of her world, and perhaps allow her to bounce or swing when she moves her feet; something portable is best, so you can move baby from room to room

○ **A bathing seat or "ring"**, which will allow her to sit upright in the tub, making bathtime an extension of the day's fun

○ **A beaker** – although she's not ready for solid foods yet, you can encourage her to start to drink from a beaker

○ **A baby toothbrush** – her teeth may not be emerging yet, but they'll be waiting under the surface, so it's a good idea to get into the habit of cleaning her gums before bedtime; you won't need toothpaste just yet

○ **A full-sized cot or bed** – most little ones will have outgrown cribs, bassinets, and baskets by this age, and will now like to have a little more space to move around

○ **Bumpers for her cot** as she starts to manoeuvre herself around more; they'll protect her from injury, and from getting stuck in the bars

○ ....

○ ....

○ ....

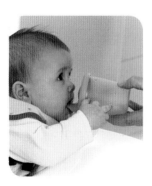 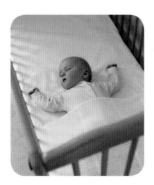 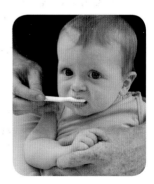

Is my baby ready for weaning?

You may find that your baby is hungrier than usual but this doesn't necessarily mean that he's ready for solid food; you may just have to up his formula intake, or allow him to suckle and feed more often.

Your baby is probably ready for solids if:

○ **He starts demanding feeds more often**, still seems hungry after his usual milk feed, and has stopped sleeping through the night

○ **He seems to show interest in what you are eating**

○ **He is able to sit up with support and control his head**

○ **He can move food around his mouth** when you feed him, or makes chewing motions even with no food in his mouth

○ **He can confidently put things into his mouth**

○ ....

○ ....

When to start

Government health authorities and the World Health Organization have now stressed that weaning should not begin before six months (although a week or two earlier won't hurt). Under no circumstances should solids be introduced until your baby is at least 17 weeks old, as a young baby's digestive and immune systems are not sufficiently developed before this time.

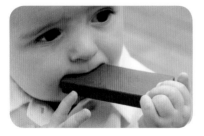

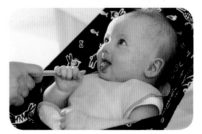

Symptoms of food allergies

Although food allergies are uncommon in babies, they are on the increase, so if you have food allergies in your family on either side, it's a good idea to be aware of the symptoms before you begin weaning your baby onto solid food. Contact your doctor if you're concerned.

Look out for:

○ **Vomiting or diarrhoea**

○ **Gagging**

○ **Irritability**

○ **Severe colic**

○ **Eczema or skin rashes** (particularly around the mouth)

○ **Hives**

○ **Facial swelling**

○ **Breathing difficulties**

Symptoms can appear while your baby is feeding, or directly after, or within 48 hours. If breathing problems develop, or his face swells, call an ambulance.

Food intolerance is slightly different, and doesn't involve your baby's immune system. It is worth looking out for symptoms suggesting that your baby can't tolerate certain foods well, as this can affect the nutrients he gets. Look out for:

○ **Chronic sniffling and excess mucus**

○ **Constipation or regular diarrhoea**

○ **Eczema or skin rashes**

○ **Unusual fatigue**

○ **Constant indigestion or possetting**

○ **Itchy eyes and skin**

○ **Sleep disturbance**

○ **Wheezing**

○ ....

○ ....

Coping with teething

Your baby may not show any signs of teething or, indeed, teeth themselves, until well into her first year of life. Some babies, however, begin teething as early as three months, so it makes sense to be prepared.

Signs of teething

○ **Irritability and fussiness**, as her gums become sore and painful; the first tooth is often the worst

○ **Drooling**

○ **Coughing or gagging**, as a result of extra saliva

○ **A rash on her chin**, mainly due to the drooling

○ **Gnawing, gumming, and biting everything** she puts in her mouth

○ **Rubbing her cheeks and pulling her ears**, as the pain travels to the ear area and around the jaw

○ **Mild diarrhoea** – this is a contentious one, as some professionals think this symptom is not linked, but a good Australian study recently found that slightly looser bowel movements are a common symptom

○ **A slightly raised temperature** – while a high fever is not a sign of teething and should be treated with caution, a low-grade fever can result from teething in some little ones; again, some doctors disagree, but parents report that it's very common

○ **Poor sleep**

○ **A runny nose**, as the ear, nose, and throat area become a little inflamed

○ _____

○ _____

It's all in the genes
The process of teething often follows hereditary patterns, so if you or your partner teethed early or late, your baby may follow the same pattern.

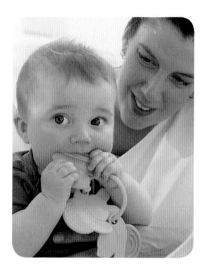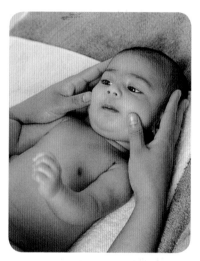

What to do

○ **Offer your baby a cool teething ring** (not one made of PVC) to gnaw on, and rub her gums with a clean finger

○ **Look for a gentle teething gel** to rub into her gums – many contain paracetamol, so take care that you don't use them at the same time as any oral doses you may be offering for pain relief

○ **The homeopathic remedy Chamomilla 30** is standard for teething, and can be taken as required up to six times a day to ease symptoms and relieve the distress; it comes in handy teething-granule form

○ **Rub a little Rescue Remedy or Emmergency Essence** into your baby's pulse points if she is crying inconsolably – a few drops at night-time will help her to sleep, as will a few drops of lavender on the bedclothes

○ **If your baby has trouble sleeping**, gentle rocking may help

○ ....

○ ....

○ ....

Childhood illnesses

Even young babies can come into contact with childhood illnesses, and experience full-blown symptoms. It can help to be aware of what your baby could catch, and what to look out for. Breastfeeding mums who are immune will likely pass on their own immunity, and if your baby has been vaccinated, he will also have some immunity of his own.

Childhood illness	Incubation period	Symptoms
Measles	10 days	Fever, runny nose, cough, sore and reddened eyes, followed by a red-brown rash that usually starts on the face and spreads down the body about 3–7 days after the first symptoms appear
Mumps	2–3 weeks	Fever, headache, swelling of the main salivary glands producing a "chipmunk" appearance affecting the jaw, cheek, and neck
Rubella (German measles)	14–21 days	A light rash of pink dots, low-grade fever, aches and pains, headaches, sore throat, swelling of lymph nodes (glands) in the neck, loss of appetite
Whooping cough (pertussis)	About 7 days	Flu-like symptoms, runny nose, sneezing, low-grade fever, a cough that worsens over a couple of weeks and is worse at night, causing paroxysms that can make your baby's face go blue or red; sometimes vomiting with coughing spells
Chickenpox	10–14 days	Headache, fever, general malaise, spots starting on the trunk and spreading to most parts of the body, appearing as little pimples that fill with fluid to form blisters that then crust over
Meningitis	Viral meningitis: 3–7 days

Bacterial meningitis: 1–7 days | Viral meningitis tends to appear most often in summer months and is generally less severe; initially vague flu-like symptoms occur with fever and aches and pains, which develop over a couple of days. Bacterial meningitis is more severe, and symptoms can develop rapidly, often within hours. In babies and small children they include: stiff body with jerky movements (or extreme floppiness), irritability or dislike of being handled, shrill cry or unusual moaning, refusal to feed, tense or bulging fontanelle, pale blotchy skin, rapid breathing, fever. In older children look for a rash that doesn't fade under pressure (try pressing a glass against the skin) |

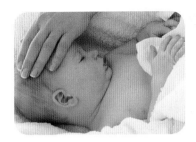

Boosting immunity

Although broadscale immunization means that most childhood illnesses are no longer prevalent, it's worth watching out for signs, and if you are worried, contact your doctor.

Treatment	Notes
Painkillers and plenty of liquids; antibiotics for any secondary infection; plenty of fluids; keep your baby in a darkened room, as measles can cause sensitivity to bright light	
Plenty of fluids, painkillers (paracetamol), rest; use tepid water to sponge your baby down	
Paracetamol to bring down the fever; calamine lotion or mild corticosteroids to ease the rash; plenty of tepid baths	
Antibiotics to clear the bacteria causing the infection; paracetamol to ease fever and discomfort; a vaporizer in the baby's environment	
Calamine lotion to ease the itching; paracetamol to reduce fever and discomfort; plenty of fluids; keep nails short and clean, or use scratch mitts	
If you suspect meningitis, you must seek emergency medical attention immediately – bacterial forms will require intravenous antibiotics; there is no treatment for viral meningitis, although medication may be offered to control the symptoms	

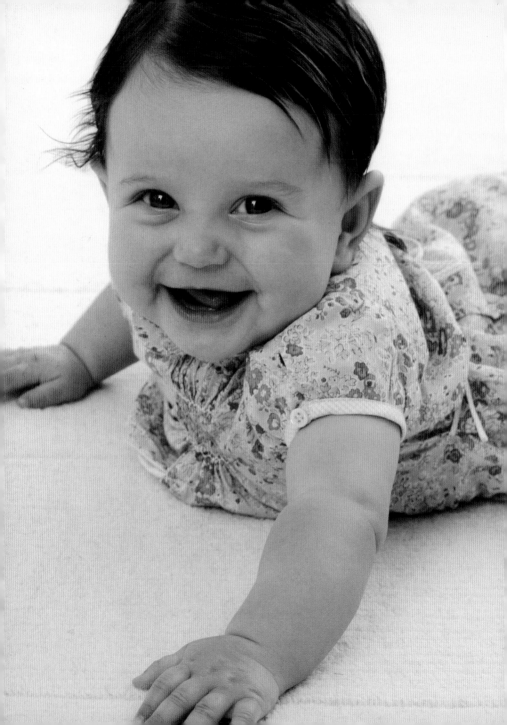

Your baby: 6–9 months

Developmental milestones

By the end of nine months, your baby will have become a sociable, lively member of the family. You'll notice a dramatic change in her development as her coordination improves, and her little brain sets to work making sense of the world around her.

By nine months, your baby should:

- ○ **Be eating solid food** along with her regular milk
- ○ **Grasp objects** on her first or second try
- ○ **See small objects easily**, and pick them up
- ○ **Move a toy easily** from hand to hand, and sit and play with toys
- ○ **Sit by herself** without pillows or other support
- ○ **Enjoy standing** when you hold her up, and begin to pull herself up to stand at the furniture
- ○ **Practise rolling** from her stomach to her back, and back again
- ○ **Begin to crawl** on her hands and knees (although some babies never crawl but develop an efficient bottom-shuffle instead)
- ○ **Move from lying down to sitting up**
- ○ **Babble and make "b" sounds**
- ○ **Enjoy blowing bubbles**
- ○ **Turn her head when you call her name**
- ○ **React positively when she sees you** – and perhaps laugh
- ○ **Search for an item** that she sees you place out of sight
- ○ **Explore everything with her mouth**
- ○ **Show signs of picking up on your emotions**, perhaps smiling when you are happy, or frowning or looking worried when you sound or look angry
- ○ **Start to imitate your actions**
- ○ **Begin to reach out to you to be picked up**
- ○ **Show the first signs of stranger or separation anxiety** (see page 184)

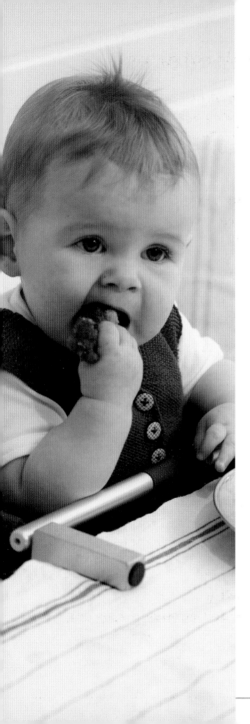

She's now ready for ...

○ **Solid food**, and in increasing amounts – by nine months she should be eating three meals a day, and beginning to show less interest in her milk feeds

○ **A firm bedtime routine**, which she will now remember and anticipate

○ **Favourite books and bedtime stories**, which she will also remember and look forward to

○ **A sturdy walker toy**, which she can use to support herself as she pulls herself up to begin the process of learning to walk

○ **Saying her first word** – she may make a sound such as "ba" that she uses, with meaning, for many different things, followed shortly afterwards by real words mixed in with the babble

○ ....

○ ....

○ ....

○ ....

○ ....

Best toys and activities

Your baby will be more mobile now, even if he hasn't yet developed the skills necessary to crawl. He'll enjoy the challenge of attempting to reach for toys and anything else that catches his interest, and his budding hand-eye coordination and motor-skill development mean that he'll become adept at playing with more sophisticated toys.

Best toys

○ **Toys that encourage crawling**, tempting your baby to follow – buy toys on a string that you pull just out of his reach, or balls that he'll chase endlessly

○ **Toys on a string** that he can pull towards him, but make sure the string is sturdy enough so it won't tangle or choke him

○ **Toys that help your baby to explore different shapes and sounds**, as well as cause and effect, shape his thinking and motor skills – try stacking toys, shape-sorters, noisy blocks, and toys that ring, rattle, and crinkle

○ **Activity boards** to help your baby to practise his coordination – he'll learn to open doors, twist, squeeze, shake, and pull things to get a reaction

○ **Blocks that can be piled** and then knocked down are always popular

○ **Containers that he can drop blocks into and then take them out** – watch him have fun with "dumping" games

○ **A sturdy walker** on which he can support his weight, pull himself up, and perhaps take a few unsteady steps

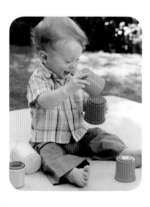 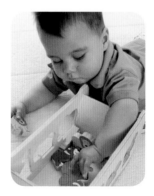 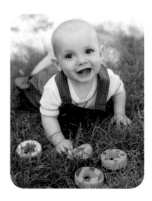

Playtime

○ **Your baby is becoming aware that objects still exist** even if he can't see them, so he'll love to play peek-a-boo and hide-and-seek games with a favourite toy

○ **Give him lots of objects to bang together**, and teach him how to play music with a pots-pans-and-wooden-spoon band

○ **Reading becomes more interactive at this age**, and he will enjoy touching the pictures, and even lifting some sturdy flaps; when you've finished reading, encourage him to turn the pages himself and "read" to you

○ **When you hear your baby babbling**, talk back to him

○ **Play simple fingers games**, such as "This little piggy" over and over and watch him delight as he anticipates the "wee wee wee all the way home"

○ **Because he is becoming better at remembering and anticipating**, any nursery rhymes or clapping games will excite him, as he looks forward to what comes next

○ **Encourage him to play on his own** (under supervision), as this will help him become independent and more confident in his own abilities

○ **Lift your baby high in the air**, or bounce him on your legs; he'll love physical games, exercise, and motion

○ _____

○ _____

○ _____

A few toys at a time

Babies can easily become overwhelmed by a huge array of toys, so bring a few out of the toy box each day, and let your baby choose what he wants to play with. You can also put a small selection of toys in a box that he can reach into and draw out what he wants.

Essential clothing and equipment

Your baby's clothing needs won't change much as she becomes more mobile, although you may wish to buy items with a little more padding to protect her knees and elbows. You will both, however, be ready for some new equipment as she forays into the world of solid food.

To wear

○ **Loose-fitting clothing** that allows your baby to move easily is the order of the day, so make sure she's dressed comfortably

○ **Three-quarter- or short-sleeved tops** will keep her hands free

○ **Look for hard-wearing clothing**, particularly at the knees

○ **Bibs are a definite necessity now**, and they should be either wipe-clean with a "tray" to collect food spills, or large and machine-washable

○ **She'll need plenty of extra changes of clothing** as she begins to experiment with food; even the very best bibs can't protect her clothes from the mess she'll create

○ **Consider a baby sleeping bag**, which fastens at the shoulders, to keep her warm in bed as she becomes adept at kicking off her covers

○ **A pair of soft rubber bootees** or an all-in-one shell suit will allow her to remain dry and comfortable while she explores the outdoor world

○ **Consider hats with under-chin fastenings**: removing and hurling hats is a popular baby game

Equipment

○ **A "jolly jumper" or a bouncing seat** that is suspended from a doorway – she may enjoy this as she becomes more confident and independent, and it will also give her legs a good work-out

○ **A toothbrush and toothpaste** – once she's eating, she'll need to have food debris cleared from her mouth twice a day, and when those teeth emerge they'll need to be brushed daily, too

○ **A foldable "umbrella" pushchair** is suitable from six months

- A **sturdy high chair** – ensure it has an insert to snugly hold a younger baby; all high chairs should have a harness or five-point belt to prevent escapes
- A **splash mat**, for under her chair
- **2–3 small plastic bowls**, preferably with a suction cup to prevent her from firing the contents across the kitchen when you least expect it
- **2–3 chunky plastic spoons** that her little hands can hold easily; she won't be able to feed herself yet, but you can encourage her to try
- **2–3 weaning spoons**, with a small "scoop" to make her first attempts at feeding a little easier
- A **plastic cup or beaker with a spout**; choose one with a "slow flow" so that she doesn't choke
- ....
- ....
- ....

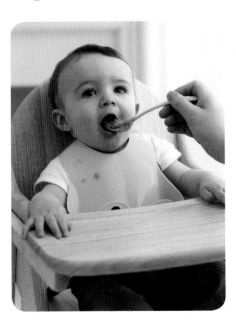

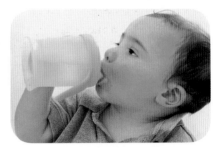

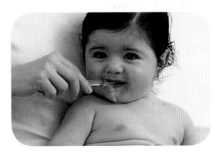

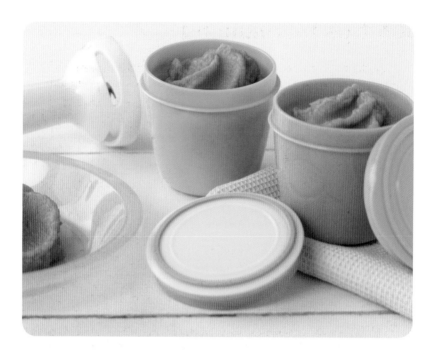

Equipment for preparing baby food

○ **A food processor** or hand-blender

○ **A hand-turned or electric grinder** (like you would use for coffee beans), which is ideal for potatoes, sweet potatoes, and other root vegetables that can become sticky and glutinous in a food processor

○ **An ice-cube tray**, which is flexible so that you can easily tip out your frozen purées; choose one with a secure lid

○ **Stick-on labels**: your purées will last for up to eight weeks in the freezer, and 24–48 hours in the fridge, so you may wish to label them with the date you made them and their contents

○ **Mini pots with lids**, to freeze larger quantities of your baby's favourites

○ ....

○ ....

○ ....

Top tips for weaning

It's important to remember that for the first few weeks of weaning, your baby will rely on his milk for nutrition and hydration. First foods are designed to accustom your baby to different tastes and textures, and encourage him to develop the skills necessary to chew (or gum) foods and swallow them.

- **First foods should be semi-liquid** and almost milk-like in consistency, to make them easy to swallow
- **Add breast milk**, formula milk, or a little cooled, boiled tap water to thin the purée if it's too thick
- **Serve him food at room temperature**, or just lukewarm – test a little on the inside of your wrist: you shouldn't feel it if it's the right temperature
- **Thoroughly defrost frozen foods**, and then warm them with a little boiled water, or in the microwave – carefully stir anything you have microwaved, as it can contain hot spots
- **Begin with some vegetables**, which aren't quite as sweet as fruit – little ones who begin with fruit tend to resist anything more savoury, and can develop a sweet tooth
- **Root vegetables are a good starter food** – try potatoes, carrots, sweet potatoes, swede, and parsnips
- **Sieve fruit and vegetables with firmer skins**, such as berries or dried fruit, to ensure that they are smooth and that there are no pips
- **Once you've established some vegetables**, blend together fruit and vegetable purées before going on to the hard stuff: pure fruit purées
- **Baby rice is also good**, and can be used to thicken purées that are too watery – make sure your baby rice is smooth and creamy
- **Encourage your baby to try some finger foods** (see page 164)
- **Offer a new food every two or three days**, and watch carefully for any signs of a reaction (see page 145), particularly if your family has food allergies; note them down in your foods diary (see page 162)
-
-

Best first foods and purées

Fruit and vegetable purées, along with baby rice and other very finely ground grains, are ideal first foods, and will not only introduce your baby to different tastes and textures, but also give her a good boost of nutrients at the same time.

Start with one-fruit or one-vegetable purées, such as:

- Baby rice
- Avocado
- Sweet potato
- Potato
- Carrot
- Parsnip
- Pumpkin
- Broad beans
- Apple
- Pear
- Banana
- Dried apricot
- Peach
- Papaya

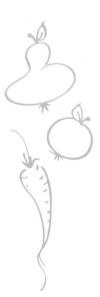

Then try some blends:

- **Root vegetables** (any blend you like)
- Carrot and squash
- Broccoli and cauliflower
- Butter beans and apple
- Pea and pear

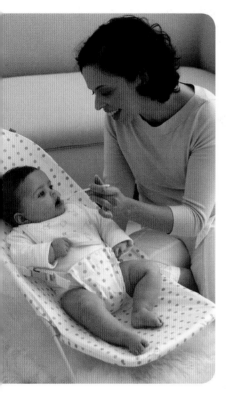

- Lentil, celery, and carrot
- Lentil and red pepper
- Spinach and potato
- Parsnip and potato
- Blueberry and melon
- Plum and pear
- Melon and mango
- Papaya and mango
- Peach and pear
- Banana and apricot
- Rice and pear
- Strawberry and banana

And when she's got the hang of it...

- Cheesy spinach and potato
- Cod, potato, and carrots
- Plaice with cheddar and parsnips
- Chicken and sweet potato
- Turkey and broccoli
- Mango and yogurt
-
-
-
-
-

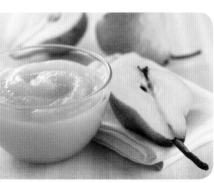

First foods diary

Jotting down what your baby eats in the early days, and noting any likes or dislikes, as well as any suspicious reactions, will form an invaluable record of her early eating habits, and make it easy to pinpoint any potential problems early on.

Food	Mixed with ...	Date offered	Likes (yes/no)	Unusual reactions (immediate/within 48 hours)

Food	Mixed with ...	Date offered	Likes (yes/no)	Unusual reactions (immediate/within 48 hours)

Great first finger foods

It's a good idea to offer finger foods alongside your baby's first purées, as they will help her to develop the skills she needs to feed herself. They'll also accustom her to different textures and tastes.

Try:

○ **Lightly steamed vegetables**, such as carrots, broccoli, and cauliflower

○ **Cucumber sticks** (with the seeds removed)

○ **Lightly toasted bread fingers**

○ **Miniature rice cakes**

○ **Very well-cooked pasta shapes**

○ **Chunks of cheese**

○ **Chunks of tuna or poached chicken**

○ **Chunks of banana**

○ **Peeled, cored apple slices or chunks of mango or pear**

○ **Dried apricots**

○ **Peach slices**

○ **Strawberries or soft blueberries**

○ **Seedless grapes**, cut in quarters to prevent choking

○ _____

○ _____

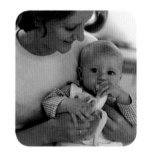

Finger foods under supervision

Watch your baby carefully while she eats finger foods, as they can cause her to gag or choke. Very first finger foods must be ones that she can gum as she won't be able to chew yet. If she does struggle, calmly remove the offending object from her mouth and pat her on the back.

Ideal family meals

It's a good idea to get your baby accustomed to eating family food from an early age, so that she learns to enjoy the taste, and also feels part of the social experience of eating as a family. Be aware, however, that salt must not be added to food intended for babies under one year of age.

Suggestions for family meals that can be puréed:

○ **Poached or steamed chicken with garden herbs** (anything goes), mashed potatoes, and green vegetables

○ **Hearty root-vegetable soup**

○ **Lightly steamed cod with spinach and new potatoes**

○ **Meatballs in a light tomato sauce with noodles or rice** – if you grind the meat finely and make small meatballs, she can eat them as finger foods

○ **Sweet potato, carrot, and ginger soup**

○ **Broccoli, leek, cauliflower, and cheese bake**

○ **Dahl** – this Indian staple will introduce her to a number of fragrant spices, and is ideal for babies if you run it through the blender first

○ **Fishcakes with avocado salad** – form her "cakes" into firm balls (make sure all of the bones are removed) before baking or lightly frying; her avocado can be puréed alongside

○ **Shepherd's pie, with a creamy mash topping**

○ **Fish pie with mashed potato topping**

○ **Oatmeal with fresh fruit purée** (give hers an extra whizz in the blender and use her usual milk to thin)

○ **Chicken and vegetable casserole**

○ **Chicken poached with apricots, sweet potato, and grapes**, and served with rice for the family

○ **Peach and apricot compôte** – serve yours with fresh yogurt, and hers with a little extra water as her own delicious dessert

○ _____

○ _____

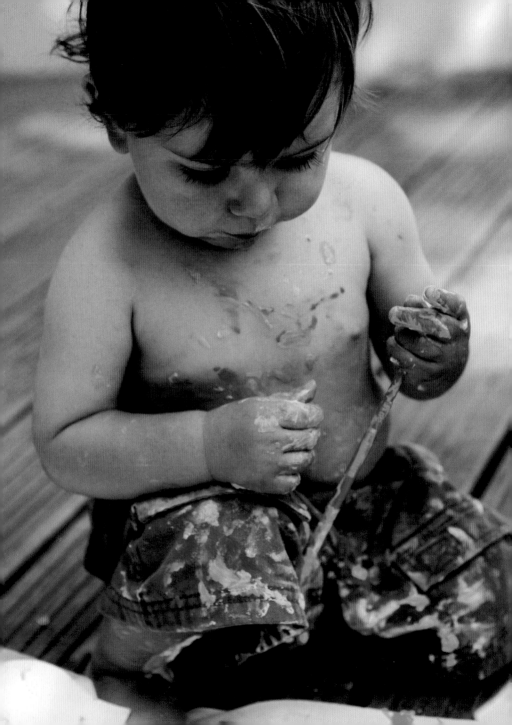

Your baby: 9–12 months

Developmental milestones

Things are happening fast now, and you may find that you are rushing to keep up with your baby as she hones her crawling skills, and manoeuvres herself around the house. Her curiosity is endless, and she now communicates with you in ways that you both understand.

By 12 months, your baby should:

○ **Confidently use a beaker**

○ **Be able to manoeuvre her spoon** to her mouth and have some success with her efforts at self-feeding

○ **Pick up toys and drop them for effect**

○ **Use her thumb and index finger** in a "pincer" grip to pick up small items

○ **Crawl confidently** forwards and backwards

○ **Pull herself up from the floor** to stand against the furniture, or you

○ **Cruise around the furniture**, supporting herself

○ **Indicate what she wants** – taking your hand if she wants a walk, or raising her arms if she wants to be held

○ **Point her finger to draw your attention to something** or show her interest

○ **Notice changes in your voice** – for example, firmness when you say "no" – and respond to her

○ **May understand the word "no"**, but probably not obey

○ **Recognize a few familiar words**, such as "bye-bye" or "milk"

○ **Recognize her name when she is called**

○ **Imitate you** – using her spoon, drinking from her cup, pretending to talk on her phone, or waving goodbye

○ **Confidently put things in and out of containers**

○ **Show an interest in pictures and books**

○ **May use the words "mama" or "dada"** appropriately

○ **Cooperate in games**

○ **Play peek-a-boo or pat-a-cake**

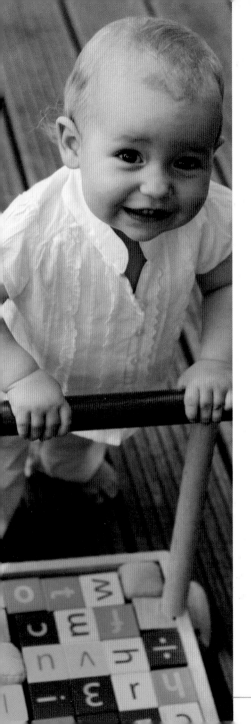

She's now ready for ...

○ **Family meals**, which she will enjoy, and which will encourage her to eat a more varied diet

○ **A new car seat**

○ **Lots of outdoor play**, for example on the swings or in the sandpit

○ **Food with more lumps** (finely chopped instead of puréed) and more exotic tastes

○ **Conversations** – she will babble back when you talk to her and pause for her reply

○ **A birthday party** ... and opening presents

○ ....

○ ....

○ ....

○ ....

○ ....

Best toys and activities

Being mobile changes your baby's world, and he will be into everything as he explores his surroundings. He'll be able to distinguish different objects, and will look for familiar toys.

Best toys

○ **Toys that your baby can push around** the room are perfect now, and he will gain speed and dexterity as he heads towards his first birthday

○ **Sorting toys, such as shape-sorters** and piles of big, chunky beads, will occupy your baby for hours

○ **Balls** continue to be popular, and he will now travel in search of a ball when it rolls away, and even try throwing it himself

○ **Water or sand tables** (or pits) will provide endless enjoyment as he fills buckets, empties them, and makes a spectacular mess

○ **Miniature versions of "adult toys"**, such as a chunky toy mobile phone, will appeal as babies begin to imitate their parents and carers at this age

○ **Interactive toys** hold new interest, and nothing will appeal to your baby more than pop-up toys and books that respond when he pushes a button

○ **Wooden or sturdy plastic blocks** or containers are ideal, and by the end of his first year he should be able to stack a few of them confidently

○ **Smaller objects to collect and a container to put them in** as he will be able to use a pincer grip effectively now

○ **Basic, sturdy wooden puzzles with knobs** to lift the pieces in and out of position will appeal – choose very simple shapes to start with

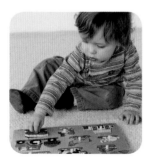 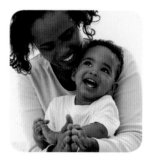 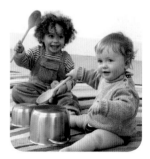

- **Toys with a string to pull** as your baby can grasp and pull quite easily now – perhaps look for a toy that climbs up its string, or makes a sound or plays a song when its string is pulled

- **Any musical toys will appeal**, and bells, maracas, and even a drum will keep him busy, and help improve his coordination and rhythm

Playtime

- **Let your baby explore and satisfy his curiosity**, opening cabinets, emptying drawers, and dumping out his toys from a basket

- **Help him to build towers**, then knock them down

- **Fill plastic tubs and shoeboxes** with toys and let him examine them, and then empty and fill the tubs again

- **When your baby points to something**, name it for him – he'll love to know the names of familiar things and it will increase his vocabulary

- **Get down on the floor and chase him** when he begins to crawl

- **Choose books that he can interact with**, and "play" with the pictures (cover the cow's eyes, for example, or ask him to tickle the pig)

- **Teach him the sounds that animals make**, and see if he can imitate them

- **Singing and dancing** is a new trick you can try – clap your hands and sing favourite nursery rhymes and encourage him to join in

- _____

- _____

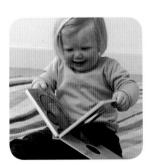
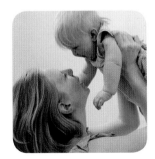
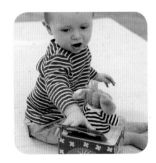

Essential clothing and equipment

The day is approaching when your little one will be ready for her first pair of shoes, and her rapid growth means that a whole host of new clothes may be necessary. She may also have outgrown some of her baby equipment, and be ready for a bigger size.

To wear

○ **Her increasing mobility means that your baby will need sturdy, washable clothes** in darker-coloured fabrics, to prevent endless piles of dirty laundry

○ **Choose clothing in complementary colours**, so that it can be easily mixed and matched and everything gets worn

○ **She'll show a new interest in being just like mum and dad**, and may like to have a pretty dress or a pair of jeans or socks just like yours

○ **She'll need three or four pairs of pyjamas without feet** – she'll enjoy using her bare feet to help her keep her balance

○ **A warm, waterproof winter jacket** is a must now, as she will escape the confines of her pushchair as often as she can and needs that extra warmth

○ **If you live in a cold climate** and winter has hit, choose mittens that attach to her coat with a plastic clip

○ **One or two pairs of rugged trousers**, such as jeans, and some comfortable sweat pants are ideal for a growing, increasingly mobile baby, no matter what the sex

○ **Team trousers with wide-necked, slip-on tops** (avoid fiddly buttons and ties because your baby won't hold still long enough to get them fastened)

○ **Non-slip socks** will help to give your baby some traction as she attempts to manoeuvre herself to her feet, or slide across the floor; let her go barefoot, too, when it's warm enough

Time to take on the stairs
Even with a stairgate your baby still needs to learn how to use the stairs – teach her to crawl up, then slide back down on her bottom, holding on to the spindles.

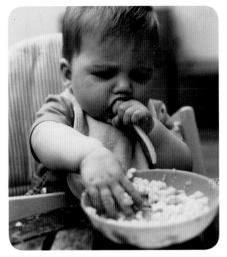
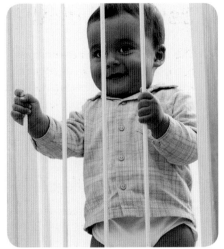

Equipment

○ **Safety equipment is essential now** – make sure you have locks on all cupboards and drawers with contents that may not be safe; you may even need a fridge lock if your little one is inquisitive

○ **Invest in a good stair gate** at the top and bottom of all flights with more than three steps

○ **Look carefully around your house and baby-proof** everything with the appropriate equipment (see page 115)

○ **Now that she's standing**, you'll want to lower the base of her cot so that she can't climb or fall out

○ **She'll be ready for her own safe, chunky cutlery set**, and will enjoy copying mum and dad

○ **A backpack-style carrier** may now make it easier to carry baby, as she grows too heavy to be carried at the front

○ **Your baby will probably be ready to graduate to the next-stage car seat** at around nine months; check the label to be sure she hasn't already outgrown the one she has

○ _____

○ _____

Your baby's first birthday

Your baby's first birthday is a momentous event, and you may wish to celebrate with a small party. Don't be surprised, though, if he doesn't show much interest in the proceedings, or if he finds the paper and the packaging more exciting than his birthday presents.

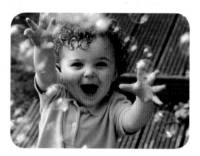

- ○ **Keep it simple** – you can't enjoy celebrating your baby's transition to toddlerhood if you are busy serving canapés

- ○ **Limit the number of guests** – most babies suffer from separation and stranger anxiety at this stage (see page 184), and a big gathering may cause distress rather than enjoyment

- ○ **Keep things short** – an hour or 90 minutes is probably the full extent of his attention span

- ○ **Set the time for the party half an hour after he normally wakes up from his nap,** so he's refreshed and not too grumpy

- ○ **Forget about themes and party games** – your baby will have no interest, and you may end up feeling deflated

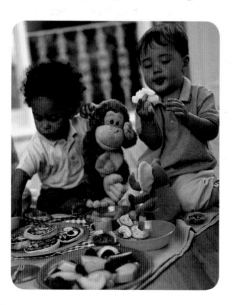

A select few
Invite only a handful of family or friends that your baby knows well, so as not to overwhelm him on his first birthday.

- **Entertainment for little ones** can be cheap and cheerful – a pot of bubbles will keep them entranced for ages

- **Balloons may be fun**, but tape them out of reach to avoid him popping them, or choking when they are deflated; better still, choose helium balloons and cut the strings so the little ones can't reach them

- **Make sure he's had something to eat and drink** before the guests arrive; even the most baby-friendly food probably won't appeal to him in the midst of all the excitement

- **Let him open his presents** – this will be the highlight of his day, if only because he will be surrounded by a mountain of crinkly, colourful paper

- **Party bags may be required for older guests**, but a shiny new ball will be enough to enthral his one-year-old buddies when they leave

- **Watch the sugar** – most little ones haven't had much experience, and can become sick and irritable on a party-food diet

- **You can make an exception to the rule** by making a wonderful, wobbly jelly, perhaps moulded in the shape of your baby's favourite animal – if you make it with half water and half fruit juice, it will have some nutritional value

- **By all means make him a cake** in the shape of something he recognizes – a farm animal, for example, or perhaps a teddy bear

- **Offer water to drink** (most baby guests will have their own cups), and some fun, healthy finger foods (see page 164)

- **If anyone asks for gift ideas, suggest books** – this is the best way to build up your baby's library, and it's an affordable gift for most people

- **If Granny and Granddad want to be more generous**, perhaps you could suggest they buy your baby his first ride-on toy, which will probably occupy him for the rest of the day

- **Don't forget your camera** – this is one day you can't fail to record

- **Take a photo of all the guests**, and tape it in your baby's scrapbook; you'll be amazed how quickly you forget his first friends, as he grows up and develops his own social circle

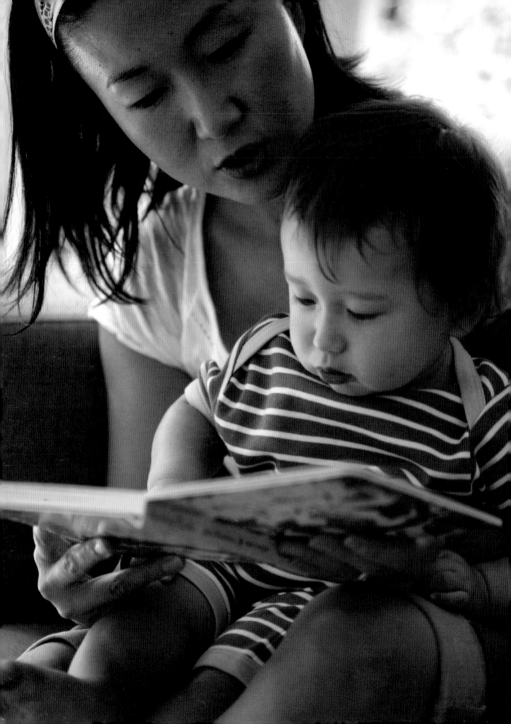

Going back to work

Preparing for your return to work

Even the most hardened career woman can't fail to feel a wrench when first leaving her baby to return to work, and circumstances may mean that you have to return earlier than you'd like. Here are some tips to help you get ready for going back to work and for coping with the first few weeks as a working mum.

- ○ **Going back to work doesn't mean you have to give up breastfeeding** – investigate whether you can have access to a quiet place to pump and a fridge for storing your milk while you are at work

- ○ **Get pumping in the weeks before you return**, and fill up your freezer – frozen breastmilk will last several months in a sealed, sterilized container

- ○ **Make sure you've got your childcare lined up** well in advance (see pages 181–183), and that you've had several trial sessions – if your baby is used to her new routine, she won't crumble when you leave for your first day back

- ○ **Make contact with your boss and colleagues** a week or two before your official return date, to touch base and get to grips with what has been going on in your absence – you'll feel more confident if you are prepared

- ○ **Bring your baby in to work a few weeks before your return**, during the lunch hour, perhaps – you'll remind colleagues of why you've been away, and give them a chance to soften when they see your beautiful baby

- ○ **Consider starting back at work on a Wednesday or Thursday**, so that you don't have a whole week to get through as soon as you are back

- ○ **Once you are back, try to stick to your schedule**; unfortunately, some workers resent women who have had time off work to have a baby, and will be looking for opportunities to prove that you can't juggle both

- ○ **Try to compartmentalize** – plan a regular phone call to your child's carer to check on things, and then get your head down and focus on your work

- ○ **Finally, take care of yourself** – juggling a baby, a household, and a job can be exhausting, so make sure you take regular breaks, drink plenty of water throughout the day, and eat well

- ○ ....

- ○ ....

- ○ ....

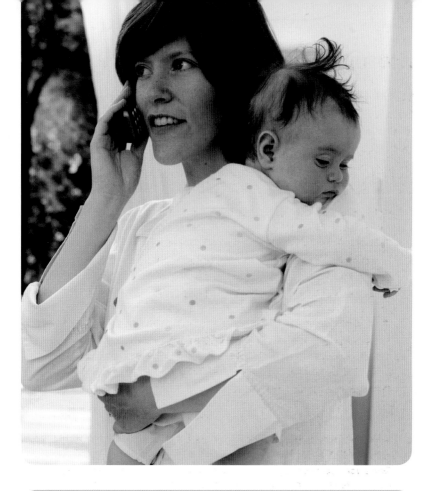

Working alternatives

Working part- or flexi-time can be the ideal solution for women who want or need to work, but who also want to spend more time with their babies in the early years. Another option is, of course, working from home. In all cases, you do need to be focused on work in the hours you've agreed, and self-disciplined enough to ensure that you achieve everything your job entails within the appropriate hours. It's all too easy to get bogged down in home and/or work life, and everyone suffers as a result. Define your hours clearly, and make sure you are doing the job of mum when you are with your baby, and career woman when you are at work.

Survival tips for working mums

It's not easy to get the balance between home and work life right, even at the best of times, and throwing a baby into the equation can make things downright difficult. There are, however, plenty of ways to ensure that you don't just survive, but thrive!

○ **Don't try to be superwoman** – you can't be perfect at everything, and if the housework slides, your baby doesn't get his bath one night, or you turn on a DVD instead of stimulating your baby, the world won't end

○ **Treat your child carer with respect** – you need her, and you need her to be happy when she is looking after your precious baby

○ **Learn to say no** – put your baby, your family, and your job at the top of the list of your priorities, and then work out what else makes sense and enhances your life; say no to anyone or anything that you don't enjoy

○ **Don't feel guilty** – many working women would choose not to work, but if that isn't an option, embrace your situation and do the best you can

○ **Take care of yourself** – an exhausted, underfed, and emotionally strung-out mum isn't any good to anyone; you'll be capable of keeping more balls in the air if you look after yourself

○ **Take care of your relationships** – your partner or husband is part of the team, too, and needs lots of love, time, and respect

○ **Always have a plan B** – things have a habit of not going to plan, and if you always have a contingency in place, life is a lot easier

○ **Establish clear guidelines at work** – you may once have been a 24-hour-a-day employee, but that is no longer possible; if everyone knows where you stand at the outset, resentment is less likely to breed

○ **Find some support in other working mums** who can be a fountain of great ideas for coping daily, and with crises; they'll also be an invaluable support network when the going gets tough

○ **Job-share at home** – make sure you divvy up the chores and the childcare, so that both you and your partner get the break you need

○ ....

○ ....

What to look for in a nursery

Places at good nurseries get booked up very quickly, and it can take some time to find the right one for you and for your baby's needs. Start looking into nurseries that might be suitable as soon as you know you are going to return to work.

Look for:

○ **A high staff-to-child ratio** – there are laws about the number of little ones that can be cared for by each responsible adult

○ **A nursery where younger and older children are separated**, meaning your baby gets the care he needs without the distractions of older kids

○ **A strong, fair discipline policy** that matches your own beliefs

○ **Permanent staff members** with good first-aid skills, as well as experience dealing with childhood illnesses and providing medical attention

○ **Well-trained staff** who constantly update their knowledge, and understand child nutrition, development, and common issues

○ **Warm, friendly, and loving staff,** who clearly show interest in the children

○ **A designated staff member for every child**

○ **A sound policy and clear evidence of safety and security**

○ **Plenty of age-related opportunities for your baby to be stimulated**

○ **A good selection of clean, tidy toys, and age-appropriate books**

○ **A quiet place for little ones to sleep**, and a clean place for them to be fed

○ **A policy of informing parents on their babies' progress daily**

○ **A good open-door policy**, so that you can visit unannounced, and feel that you are welcome at any time

○ **A glowing inspection report**, or several very good personal references: ask around – other parents won't lie

○ **Above all, trust your instinct** – if you see contented babies and warm, caring staff, you are probably on to a good thing

○ _____

○ _____

Finding the right nanny

It can be quite daunting to hand over your baby to someone else to look after, and you will need to develop a close relationship with your child's carer. Take the time to interview prospective nannies well in advance, then go with your gut feelings: they are almost always right.

○ **Draw up a full job description**, involving every aspect of your baby's day-to-day care, and what you'd like to see happening

○ **Write this down in a bullet-pointed list**, so you can talk through each aspect and issue and get feedback, ideas, and opinions

○ **Make sure you have your baby in tow at interviews** – prospective nannies should be interested, playful, and affectionate with her

○ **Check that she has emergency first-aid training** and ask to see her childcare certifications, diplomas, and driving licence

○ **Take up at least two personal and two professional referees**

○ **Her basic knowledge of and views on child development** should be up to date and consistent with yours

○ **She should have plenty of ideas for stimulating your baby**

○ **She should share your approach to nutrition and meal planning**, or be prepared to adopt it

○ **She should absolutely share your views on discipline**

○ **Organizational skills are essential**, and she should be able to keep track of everything in your little one's daily life

○ **Ask where she sees herself in five years' time** – continuity of care is important to small children

○ **Ask for details of her strengths and weaknesses**, and be wary if she says she has none of the latter

○ **Make sure she's flexible**, and won't mind working longer hours from time to time, or planning some of her holidays when you have yours

○ _____

○ _____

○ _____

What to look for in a childminder

Having your baby looked after in someone else's home is often a good solution to the childcare dilemma, and your little one will benefit from the company of a small group of other children. Look for:

○ **A registration certificate, a good Ofsted inspection report, and references** from other parents

○ **Not too many children** – there are laws outlining how many children of each age can be cared for, and it's important that this is maintained

○ **A cheerful, friendly demeanour**, and an obvious interest in children

○ **Someone with plenty of ideas**, willingly outlined, for stimulating your baby and keeping tabs on her development

○ **A clean, welcoming, smoke-free home**, with an outdoor play area

○ **A policy on TV viewing that matches your own**

○ **Knowledge and experience of first aid**

○ **A similar approach to yours to discipline, potty training, and nutrition**

○ **A willingness to enter into a contract** that outlines hours, sick pay, what happens when your child is ill, changes to your child's routine, and payment

○ **Flexibility**, so if you are running late or have an early start, you are covered

○ ....

○ ....

Keeping track
Ask your carer to write down some notes each day about what your baby did, including what she ate, what she played with, when she slept and for how long, and any milestones she may have reached.

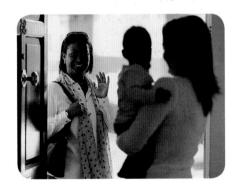

Soothing separation anxiety

Separation anxiety normally rears its head at about six months of age, when your baby has developed a strong attachment to you as his primary carer. There are, however, plenty of ways to ease the pain of separation, and make the experience more positive for you both.

○ **Don't go out of your way to avoid separations** when your baby is young – he should get used to being with other people

○ **You can try to leave the room** for a couple of seconds at a time, and then reappear – this will help him learn from a young age that you will always return after you go away

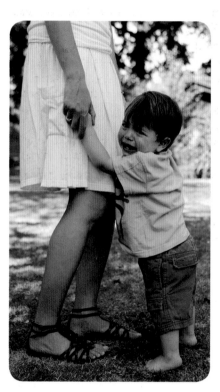

Be kind to yourself

Bear in mind that guilt is a destructive emotion, and can undermine your self-confidence and even your relationship with your baby. All mums suffer from "bad-mother syndrome" from time to time. Accept that this is par for the course, and then make a conscious effort to pat yourself on the back for managing to juggle so many areas of your life. You are doing the best you can and most likely you are doing a wonderful job, so make sure you acknowledge that, and believe in the fact that both you and your baby are capable of being happy and fulfilled with a working-mum lifestyle.

○ **Introduce new babysitters (and carers) gradually,** letting your baby get to know them before being left alone with them

○ **Provide transitional objects,** such as a favourite teddy or blanket, which your baby will use to cope with separation; leaving behind a scarf or T-shirt with your scent firmly embedded can also help to ease the transition

○ **Try not to make light of your baby's distress** – comfort him and reassure him; tell him you know he is sad and reassure him that you love him and you will be back soon

○ **Always say goodbye** – disappearing will make your baby feel insecure; if you say goodbye, he'll soon understand that this means you are leaving and he'll also start to remember that you always come back

○ **Don't be surprised if your baby needs lots of reassurance** before and after separations – spend some time offering just that

○ **Show plenty of warmth and approval for your carer** – if your baby knows you are comfortable with her, he will feel that much happier in her care

○ **Talk it up** – show pleasure and excitement that you are going to the nursery, or that your carer is about to arrive; if you are positive about the experience, your baby will pick up the right signals and soon follow suit

○ **Similarly, try not to cry or appear anxious** – if he senses something is wrong, your baby may become even more distressed; you have to go to work, and he will have a wonderful, fulfilling, fun time while you are gone

○ **Try as much as possible to return on time** – if you don't turn up when your baby expects you to (if you always bathe him, for example, or always give him a night-time feed), he may become anxious and distrustful

○ **Remember that you can suffer from separation anxiety, too** – reassure yourself that you have chosen a good, reliable carer that you trust, and that your baby will be safe and happy with her

○ --

○ --

○ --

Covering holidays and illness

Even the most carefully set up childcare arrangements can fall to pieces from time to time, when your baby or your carer is ill, or your carer takes a holiday. It's a good idea to have contingency plans set up in advance for emergencies, and to help get you through periods when no one is available to hold the baby.

○ **All children fall ill**, and babies and very young children are particularly susceptible because of their immature immune systems – make sure you are aware of any sickness policies at your nursery, crèche, or childminder

○ **Remember, too, that all carers are entitled to holidays** (and holiday pay), so it's a good idea to establish at the outset when holidays may take place

○ **Check with your employer** to establish what their policy is about taking time off when your children are ill, so you know what to expect – you may be required to use up your personal sick days

○ **You might be able to arrange to work at home** when your child is ill – it's a good idea to establish remote access with your work computer, and to have some work ready that you can get on with if you can't get into the office

○ **Working at home is a good option for longer periods of illness**, or for holiday cover for your carer; perhaps a friend's au pair or mother's help can work for you for some of the day to help make sure you get your work done

○ **In the UK you are entitled to emergency family leave**, which stipulates a "short amount of unpaid time off" – but just because it's law doesn't mean that your employer and colleagues are going to be happy when you take it

○ **See if you can take turns with your partner to care for your child**

○ **Set up a bank of family members or friends** who can step in at short notice

○ **Ask another mum in advance** if she would be prepared to share her nanny or au pair to help you out in a pinch – you could offer the same in return, or something similar, such as an evening's babysitting

○ **Establish a strong support network** both at work and with any other mums at your child's childcare facility – it's easier to arrange swaps and ask for favours if you are on a first-name basis

○ **Try not to feel guilty about asking for favours**; we are all conditioned to think that asking for help is a sign of weakness, but working mums need all the help they can get

- **Be honest with your work colleagues** – they'll appreciate the fact that you are up-front about your position, and probably be only too glad to help out

- **Check out agency workers in advance** – you will have to pay for having a carer at short notice, but it can save you a lot of hassle and concern

- **Plan for your carer's holidays in advance** by arranging short-term cover – a gap-year student or someone from your local childcare college may be only too glad to earn some extra money and get some experience

- **Join a time bank** – you can put in hours helping someone with their accounts, or even babysitting, and "earn" them back in childcare hours

- **Consider arranging your own holidays** when your carer is taking a break; you'll remove the pressure of finding cover, and you'll enjoy the experience of sharing time as a family

- _____

- _____

- _____

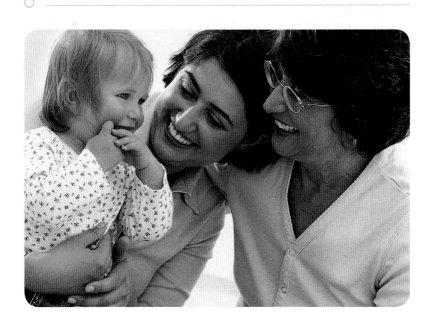

Staying at home

Staying at home with your baby may seem like a luxury to some, but it may well be the hardest job you'll ever do. However, every ounce of patience spent and every nerve frayed will result in the most rewarding experience of your life.

○ **It goes without saying that it should be financially feasible** – if staying at home is going to send you into massive debt and put enormous pressure on your family relationships, you may need to rethink

○ **Try living on one salary** for a couple of months before or just after your baby is born, putting any maternity pay you receive in a savings account – if you can manage, then give it a whirl

○ **Consider the benefits you may lose, too** – if you depend on employer pension contributions, healthcare benefits, and your company car, there might be more of a financial hole than you had thought

○ **Find out which benefits your partner can get through his job** – it might be more cost-effective for your partner to stay at home with the baby

○ **Make sure you establish a good network of other mums with babies** – not only is the stimulation important for you both, but you'll be party to a wealth of shared ideas, concerns, and wisdom

○ **Make sure your partner appreciates your efforts** and takes some responsibility for the household chores, too; don't feel you have to be superwoman – your priority is your baby's health and wellbeing

○ **Take time out to read the paper** and to get the housework and shopping done – little ones do need to grow up understanding that there are other things that require mum's or dad's attention from time to time

○ **Keep up with courses or activities that will keep your work skills sharp,** so that if you do go back to work you'll be ready

○ ....

○ ....

○ ....

Index

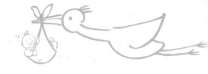

Useful websites

Birth options

○ www.aims.org.uk (Association for Improvements in Maternity Services)
www.babycaretens.com
www.birthchoiceuk.com
www.gentle-birth.net
www.homebirth.org.uk
www.hypnobirthing.co.uk
www.independentmidwives.org.uk
www.tens-hire.co.uk
www.waterbirth.co.uk

Breastfeeding advice

○ www.abm.me.uk (Association of Breastfeeding Mothers)
www.breastfeedingnetwork.org.uk
www.laleche.org.uk
National Breastfeeding Helpline:
0844 20 909 20
www.nct.org.uk
NCT breastfeeding line: 0870 444 8708

Childbirth classes

○ www.nctpregnancyandbabycare.com
www.activebirthcentre.com

Childcare

○ www.ofsted.gov.uk

Eco-friendly baby nursery

○ www.mylittleeco.co.uk
www.spiritofnature.co.uk
www.alotoforganics.co.uk

Natural remedies

○ www.victoriahealth.com
www.nealsyardremedies.com

Reusable nappies

○ www.twinkleontheweb.co.uk
www.thenappylady.co.uk
www.kittykins.co.uk.

Acknowledgments

Author's Acknowledgments

The author would like to thank Peggy Vance, Penny Warren, and Helen Murray at DK for coming up with a great idea, and pushing to make sure it happened. Thanks to Angela Baynham and Helen for excellent editing and ideas, and Hannah Moore and Liz Sephton for a lovely design. I'm also grateful to the National Childbirth Trust, Annabel Karmel, and AIMS for information, as well as to homeopath and hynotherapist Melanie Woollcombe. New mums Karol Allen and Erica Manger made sure I got it spot on, and have tried and tested the checklists for accuracy. Finally, thanks to my own little one, Marcus, and the older two, Cole and Luke, who gave me the experience I needed to write this book.

Publisher's Acknowledgments

DK would like to thank Hilary Bird for the index, Salima Hirani for proofreading, and Lizzie Ette for checking the information in the book.

Picture Credits

The publisher would like to thank the following for their kind permission to reproduce their photographs:

Corbis: image100 71 (left); Mother & Baby Picture Library: Ian Hooton 112 (left)

All other images © Dorling Kindersley

For further information see:
www.dkimages.com